DEBRA WATERHOUSE, M.P.H., R.D.

THE NATIONAL BESTSELLER

OUTSMARTING

THE FEMALE

FAT CELL

THE FIRST WEIGHT-CONTROL PROGRAM DESIGNED *SPECIFICALLY* FOR WOMEN

WARNER BOOKS 60129-2 $5.99 U.S.A. ($6.99 CAN.)

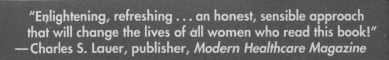

"Enlightening, refreshing . . . an honest, sensible approach that will change the lives of all women who read this book!"
—Charles S. Lauer, publisher, *Modern Healthcare Magazine*

0-446-60129-2-00599-3

9 780446 601290

50599

DO YOU NEED TO STOP DIETING AND START EATING?

Rate each of the following statements as follows:

0—Never, 1—Seldom, 2—Frequently, 3—Always

1. I count calories. _____
2. I'm either on a diet or off a diet. _____
3. I eat diet foods. _____
4. I feel out of control with food. _____
5. Dieting is more important than good nutrition. _____
6. I start my diets on Monday. _____
7. I eat for emotional reasons. _____
8. Hunger is a foreign feeling to me. _____
9. I wait until I am extremely hungry before I eat. _____
10. I eat to prevent hunger. _____

If you scored 15 or more points, *Strategy #2* will help you give up dieting once and for all. It will teach you how to eat again. It's one of the six savvy strategies that shows you how to start . . .

OUTSMARTING THE FEMALE FAT CELL

DEBRA WATERHOUSE is a nationally known and respected nutrition expert and speaker in the areas of weight control, eating disorders, fitness, cancer, and women's nutrition issues. More than twenty thousand women have attended her seminars and workshops. She lives and works in the San Francisco Bay area.

Please turn this page for endorsements from experts for *Outsmarting the Female Fat Cell*

OUTSMARTING
THE FEMALE
FAT CELL

DEBRA WATERHOUSE, M.P.H., R.D.

WARNER BOOKS

A Time Warner Company

The programs in this book are not intended for persons with chronic illnesses or other conditions that may be worsened by an unsupervised eating program or exercise program. The recommendations are not intended to replace or conflict with advice given to you by your physician or other health-care professionals, and we recommend that you do consult your physician.

WARNER BOOKS EDITION

Copyright © 1993 by Debra Waterhouse, M.P.H., R.D.
All rights reserved.

Cover design by Tom Radom
Cover photograph by Ron Puhlaski

This Warner Books Edition is published by arrangement with Hyperion, 114 Fifth Avenue, New York, New York 10011.

Warner Books, Inc.
1271 Avenue of the Americas
New York, NY 10020

Visit our Web site at
http://pathfinder.com/twep

 A Time Warner Company

Printed in the United States of America

First Warner Books Printing: May, 1994

10 9

To my parents
Alina and Ray Waterhouse
whose infinite love and encouragement
provided the spirit and confidence
to achieve this goal
and all others in my life

First Warner Books Printing: May, 1994

switches them on. You already know about the effects of estrogen, but let me summarize so that you can view the whole

Acknowledgments

■

THE TWO most important people in my life, my husband and my sister, have been by my side from the first flickering idea to the final manuscript. They deserve much more than acknowledgment—they deserve the medal of unsurpassed honor.

To my patient husband, Paul Manca, who has not only been my most truthful critic, but also my most enduring companion. You were my emotional stabilizer and my reality checker. Only you could have played that important role.

To my beautiful sister, Lori Waterhouse Erwin, for her infinite support, encouragement, and love. What would I have done without you?

I am forever indebted to Cynthia Traina, of Traina Public Relations in San Francisco, who provided the first sign of hope that I could become a writer and who passed along a name that would change my life, Sandra Dijkstra.

A million thanks to my agent, Sandra Dijkstra, and her associate, Katherine Goodwin Saideman, who went above and beyond the call of duty. Your expertise, reputation, and commitment made it all happen.

In a society driven by fad diets and quick weight-loss schemes, my editor, Judith Riven, and all at Hyperion had the unquestionable belief in me and in my approach. Thank you for making my dream a reality.

There are so many other friends, colleagues, and family

members (yes, that includes you, Laura Euphrat) who also deserve acknowledgment for their creative input and their listening ears. I'm sure that you have been bored to tears with my incessant preoccupation with this project. Thank you for being there for me.

Contents

■

OUTSMARTING

THE FEMALE

FAT CELL

treams, and permanently changes the physiology of your
fat cells by switching them off." As you will discover, this

Why You Should Read This Book

■

I F YOU are in search of a revolutionary, honest, scientifically sound, fat-fighting program designed specifically for women—look no further, you've found it! It's called the **OFF** Plan:

O	F	F
U	E	A
T	M	T
S	A	
M	L	
A	E	
R		
T		
I		
N		
G		

What you are about to encounter is *not* a diet. A diet is a restrictive reduction of calories that is virtually impossible to follow for more than a month and that is often psychologically and physiologically devastating. The **OFF** Plan is the direct opposite of a diet: It is a realistic approach to changing habits that allows you to eat whatever you want, lasts a lifetime, and permanently changes the physiology of your fat cells by switching them "off." As you will discover, the

OFF Plan has nothing to do with dieting and everything to do with eating. It is a refreshing, delicious alternative to dieting.

Years ago, when I first started my nutrition counseling practice, I immediately became aware of the drastic differences in weight loss between men and women. I was perplexed as to why my female clients lost less weight and lost it more slowly. Over the past couple of years, fascinating research has been conducted that proves what I had already suspected (and you probably suspected too)—female fat cells are physiologically different from male fat cells. They are smart, stubborn, love to store fat, and hate to give it up.

The world's leading obesity researchers have discovered that a woman's fat cell is bigger because it has more fat-*storing* enzymes, while a man's fat cell is smaller because it has more fat-*releasing* enzymes. Studies done at Cedars-Sinai Medical Center in Los Angeles and other research facilities have found that a woman's hip and thigh fat cells are at least twice as efficient in storing fat and enlarging than they are in releasing fat and shrinking. It's no wonder that men tend to lose weight quickly and keep it off, while women tend to lose weight slowly and gain it back. When it comes to dieting, a woman's fat physiology works against her.

What makes a woman's fat cell different from a man's? I can answer this question in one word—estrogen. Estrogen "feeds" the fat cells in the hips, buttocks, and thighs. It protects the fat cell by making it extremely efficient at storing fat. A woman's fat cell needs this special protection because it has special functions that a man's fat cell does not; it needs to store as many calories as possible to ensure fertility and pregnancy. This protection starts during puberty when the initial surge of estrogen causes adolescent girls to accumulate fat in the hips and thighs. During pregnancy, as you may have experienced, those fat cells store like crazy to protect the growing fetus. Researchers at Johns Hopkins and elsewhere have found that when women receive some additional estrogen through oral contraceptives or estrogen replacement therapy, there is also an increase in body fat. I think that the most convincing studies have been done with men. When men are given estrogen, they quickly gain hip and thigh fat— and have a difficult time losing it!

You deserve to know, understand, and acknowledge the medical fact that a woman's hormones and fat physiology make it more difficult for her to achieve weight loss. Even more importantly, you deserve the special attention necessary to finally be successful at weight control.

This book has two major purposes:

1. To provide an understanding of how your female fat cells function.
2. To provide the solution to permanently outsmarting your female fat cells and achieve a comfortable weight.

I'm sure that you are saying to yourself: "This sounds great, but how much weight will I lose on the OFF Plan?"

I will not make false promises for the purpose of book sales and temporary fame. I will not guarantee "a pound a day," "three pounds a week," "twenty pounds a month." Women are simply not equipped with the fat-burning machinery necessary to lose weight this quickly and keep it off. I don't want you to buy this book with the hope that it is this month's answer to losing the excess fifteen pounds. It is, however, your physiology's answer to outsmarting your female fat cells forever.

I will not make promises that I cannot keep. But here is what I *can* promise you:

- You will lose as much weight as is realistically and genetically possible for you.
- You will never have to diet again.
- You will learn to eat whatever you desire without guilt and without gaining weight.
- You will gain an understanding of your body, your fat cells, and your physiology.
- You will work with your female physiology (not against it) to outsmart your fat cells.

- You will gain peace of mind, knowing that you are not a failure at the weight-loss battle.
- You will never have to count calories again.
- You will never have to give up any favorite foods.
- You will develop a healthy relationship with food.
- You will transform your fat-storing body into a fat-burning body.
- You will permanently shrink your fat cells with special eating and exercise guidelines developed for a woman's body.

So, to answer the key question, "How much weight will I lose?," you will lose as much as you want to on the OFF Plan as long as your goal is realistic. Because of society's pressure for thinness, most women are striving for the "perfect" body projected by Madison Avenue ad-makers, one that is not biologically possible for them to achieve. If your goal is unrealistic and virtually unobtainable, you will never be successful. Realistic goals take into consideration age, genetics, reproductive history (pregnancies, method of contraception, menopause, estrogen replacement, and other factors), body fat, and body type. I'll help you to set realistic goals.

Now the second question, "How fast will I lose the weight I want to lose?," is a more difficult question to answer. I do not promise or advocate quick weight loss. It is a well-documented fact that the more quickly you lose the weight, the more quickly you gain it back. I can, however, give you some realistic expectations for safe, permanent weight loss based on my experience with over 200 clients.

Before presenting what I have learned from evaluating my clients over the years, I need to give you some background. "Real" weight loss is fat loss. Reducing the pounds of fat on your body by reducing the size of your fat cells is the ultimate goal. You do not want to lose muscle mass. Muscle is metabolically active tissue that burns fat and calories. On the contrary, I encourage you to gain muscle through exercise. The more muscle mass you have, the faster your metabolism, the more you can eat, and the more fat you will lose. One of the major reasons athletes can eat more and weigh less is because of their increased muscle mass, but you do not have to be a marathon runner to get this benefit. Gaining a couple of pounds of muscle will not make you a bigger person. Muscle is dense tissue and weighs more than fat. You can lose one pound of fat and gain one pound of muscle—and become a smaller person.

The bathroom scale does not tell you how much muscle and fat you have, how much fat you have lost, and how much muscle you have gained. This is why I will advise you to throw away your scale and instead have your body composition analyzed. Body composition analysis separates your fat weight from your muscle weight and tells you what is inside your body. In the following analysis of my clients, the pounds of muscle gained and fat lost were calculated from body-composition analysis using skinfold calipers. Calipers are used by health professionals to measure the amount of fat under the arm (the sagging fat that prevents us from wearing sleeveless tops), the hips, the thighs, and other areas.

The OFF Plan Results

	NUMBER OF MONTHS				
	1	**3**	**6**	**9**	**12**
Pounds of fat lost	2	8	11	15	21
Pounds of muscle gained	1	3	4	5	5
Pounds of weight lost	1	5	7	10	16
Inches lost in waist	0.5	1.5	2.5	4.0	6.5
Inches lost in hips	0.2	1.0	2.0	3.5	6.0
Inches lost in thighs	0.2	0.5	1.5	2.0	3.0

You may be looking at these results with great disappointment—lose one pound in one month, five pounds in three months—Forget it! If you look instead at the pounds of fat lost and the inches lost, these numbers are actually quite encouraging. The average pounds of fat lost is eight pounds in three months and twenty-one pounds in one year. If you look at the inches lost in the waist, hips, and thighs, you'll discover the body size is smaller because of reduced fat and increased muscle mass.

Fat cells cannot be fooled overnight, within a week, or even within a month. I recommend that women give themselves three months to see noticeable changes in their bodies and to have a realistic time frame in achieving their ultimate goals with the OFF Plan. Any program that promises immediate results is not going to permanently change the physiology of your fat cells and has profit, not your long-term success and well-being, as its motive.

Now for the third question, "Will I gain the weight back?" If you make the OFF Plan a natural part of your lifestyle, you will not gain the weight back. A natural part of your lifestyle is the key phrase in guaranteeing long-term success. The OFF Plan must be compatible with every aspect of your professional and private lives. The Plan must be able to change as your lifestyle changes.

The OFF Plan is not a three-week meal plan to follow (you'll be happy to hear that there are no meal plans at all), or a liquid drink you consume every day for lunch, or a list of mandatory changes that each of you has to follow. These alternatives are not natural, lifestyle changes because you cannot practice them for the rest of your life. This is why many of the commercial weight-loss programs have such low long-term success rates—at best only 5 to 10 percent keep the weight off. The OFF Plan has an 80 percent one-year success rate and a 62 percent five-year success rate. You are about ten times more likely to keep the weight off with the OFF Plan.

The OFF Plan is a natural, lifestyle approach to permanently changing the physiology of your female fat cells. It includes 6 effective strategies that are scientifically based and the result of my eight years' experience in helping thousands of women to outsmart their fat cells.

STRATEGY #1: Aerobicize Your Fat Cells
STRATEGY #2: Stop Dieting and Start Eating
STRATEGY #3: Feed Your Body, Not Your Fat Cells
STRATEGY #4: Shrink and Multiply Your Meals
STRATEGY #5: Become a Daytime Eater
STRATEGY #6: Fat-Proof Your Diet

The 3-month **OFF** Plan will give you guidance on how to make these strategies a part of your life—how to get started, how to set and achieve goals, and how to monitor your progress. Unlike a rigid diet plan (where you are either on the diet or off the diet) the **OFF** Plan is flexible, sensible, and lasts a lifetime. Eventually, it stops being a "plan" and becomes the way you are.

This book is divided into three important phases:
1. Chapters 1 through 3 will give you the knowledge and understanding of how your female fat cells function.
2. Chapters 4 and 5 will prepare you for a successful program by enhancing your readiness and commitment. They will help you to:

   • think in terms of permanent weight loss, not temporary weight loss
   • think in terms of slow weight loss, not quick weight loss
   • think in terms of body fat, not weight loss

3. The remaining chapters will provide the step-by-step **OFF** Plan and all the skills you need to outsmart your female fat cells forever.

Forget dieting, forget calories—and begin a new natural and sensible way of eating that works within the realities of a woman's body, not against it.

Now, are you ready to outsmart your female fat cells? Watch out fat cells, here we come!

Chapter One

■

YOU CAN'T COMPARE
APPLES AND PEARS

WHEN I first started my practice, a couple came to see me for support in losing weight. They were both about twenty pounds overweight and thought that it would be a little easier and a lot more fun to lose weight together. I put them on an exercise program and helped them make some positive changes in their eating habits. A month went by, the man lost seven pounds, the woman gained one pound. When I asked if there were any differences in what they were doing, the answer was no. They were eating the same types of foods and walking together. Another month went by—the man lost another six pounds and the woman lost one pound (the pound she gained in the first month). She was frustrated, depressed, and ready to give up exercise for chocolate. I was just as perplexed and frustrated, and ready to give up my practice.

It was then that I realized how different men and women really are and became interested in the mysterious female fat cell.

So, I did some research on women's fat metabolism and discussed with the couple the reality that men were born with the fat-burning machinery to lose weight more quickly than women. I asked the wife if I could do some experimentation, change her exercise program a bit and modify her eating habits. Two months later she was catching up with her husband, and within six months they had both reached their goals.

The fact is that women are different from men—a difference that goes way beyond the obvious to the internal composition of the body. The female fat cell is large, powerful, and stubborn—and explains why women lose less weight, lose it more slowly, and gain it back more quickly than men.

However, before we can understand how the female fat cell can sabotage our efforts at weight control, we must first investigate what a fat cell is and how it works.

You have over 30 billion fat cells (yes, 30 *billion*) in your body right now that are capable of storing 150-plus pounds of fat. A fat cell's sole purpose is to store calories when you do not need them and to release calories when you do need them. There are names for the storage and release of fat:

lipogenesis = the storage of fat
"lipo' means fat/"genesis" means formation

lipolysis = the release of fat
"lipo" means fat/"lysis" means breakdown

A fat cell does not function alone; it requires help from a complex enzyme system. Enzymes facilitate the transport of fat in and out of the fat cell. It's no surprise that the enzymes that help store fat are called the *lipogenic* enzymes, and the enzymes that help release fat are the *lipolytic* enzymes.

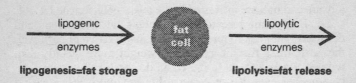

lipogenic enzymes → fat cell → lipolytic enzymes

lipogenesis=fat storage   **lipolysis=fat release**

Both men and women have about the same number of fat cells, but that's where the similarities end. The major difference between male and female fat cells is in the enzyme systems and the size of the fat cells. You guessed it! Women have more lipogenic enzymes for the storage of fat, and the more you can store, the bigger the fat cell. Men have more lipolytic enzymes for the release of fat and, therefore, have smaller fat cells.

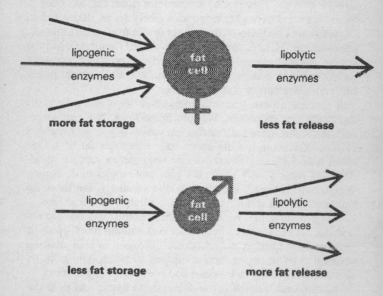

Simply stated, women have what it takes to store fat quickly and efficiently. Men have what it takes to release fat quickly and efficiently. Women lose fat very slowly; men store fat very slowly. If you are wondering why women got the fat end of the deal, the answer has to do with the reason why women are women. Estrogen, the female sex hormone, activates and multiplies the lipogenic enzymes. This explains the increase in body fat during puberty, pregnancy, and when women are taking oral contraceptives or estrogen replacement therapy. Mother Nature had a purpose in making us the fatter sex: Women need more fat to be healthy, stay fertile and bear children. You can't be a woman without some fat.

Estrogen not only stimulates the lipogenic enzymes to store fat but also directs where most of the fat will be stored. This is another major difference between men and women. Estrogen concentrates its fat-storing efforts in the buttocks, hips, and thighs. The average woman has a size-8 top and a size-12 bottom. This is why women are often called "pears." When men gain weight, it is more likely to be deposited in the waist area because of the effects of the male sex hormone, testosterone. Hence, men are often called "apples." Maybe apples and oranges are not the only fruits you can't compare. Based on these gender differences in fat cells, you definitely can't compare apples and pears either.

If you are a pear, you will gain weight first and take it off last in the hips and thighs. Fat cells in the lower body are larger and have more lipogenic-storing enzymes. If you go on a diet or start exercising, it's the upper body that loses fat first. One client was ready to give up exercise because her smaller shoulders and breasts only made her hips and thighs look bigger. Weight will come off the lower body eventually, but those fat cells are resistant and it may take longer than you would like.

If you're an apple, which does run in some families, the abdominal fat cells tend to be smaller and contain more lipolytic enzymes for quicker weight loss. Estrogen is still making your fat cells stubborn, but, compared to pears, you may respond more quickly to exercise and positive eating habits.

As men and women grow older, these apple and pear descriptions become even more apparent. To visualize this with some humor, one of my clients shared a little joke: "As men grow older they get Dunlop's disease because the belly 'dun lops' over the belt. As women grow older, they get Furniture's disease because the chest eventually falls into the drawers." Oh well, so much for humor.

Let me give you an example of how all of this female fat physiology works in a real-life situation. You've had a tough day, you're overhungry, and you devour a fourteen-inch pepperoni pizza for dinner. Your body needs some of these calories (maybe three slices' worth) to function, but the remaining five slices are excess calories traveling around in your bloodstream that your body doesn't need. Because your hip and thigh fat cells have the greatest ability for storage, those extra five slices are transported into those fat cells by the lipogenic enzymes. You now have bigger hip and thigh fat cells even before the chocolate ice cream dessert.

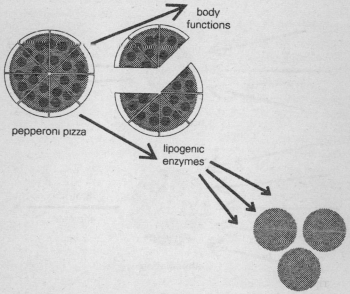

body functions

pepperoni pizza

lipogenic enzymes

hip and thigh fat cells

Our bodies' efficiency at storing fat goes beyond the fact that we are women with estrogen. Because of our frustration with weight loss, we have become professional dieters. I have yet to find a woman who has never been on a diet, and most women attempt at least two diets a year.

Dieting, as you will discover in Chapter 2, is the female fat cell's best friend. If women knew what dieting really does to their bodies, they would never, ever, even think about the new diet they plan to start on Monday. As soon as your fat cells realize that calories have been reduced, they throw a party and invite the lipogenic enzymes to store fat. Unfortunately, lipolytic enzymes are not on the guest list. Dieting simply increases the size of your fat cells, improves your body's ability to store fat, and limits your ability to burn it.

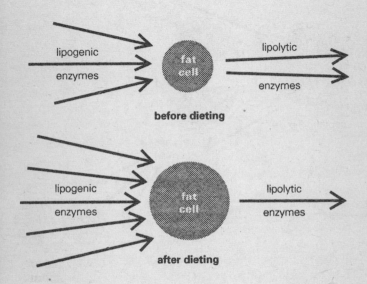

Since we are comparing apples and pears, a man's fat cells react differently to dieting; they do not share these same fat-storing effects. When men go on a traditional diet, they have the fat-burning machinery to lose weight and keep it off—as a matter of fact, they are twice as likely to keep the weight off. When women go on a traditional diet, they may lose weight, but then they gain it back plus some.

I must mention one more difference between men and women: the muscle cell. It's not that male and female muscle cells function differently; it's that men have more muscle cells—about 40 percent more. Muscle contains special calorie-burning structures called "mitochondria" that converts calories to heat and water. So, when it comes to the decision on where calories go in the body, the more muscle cells you have, the more calories are directed to the muscle cells to be burned and the less to the fat cells to be stored.

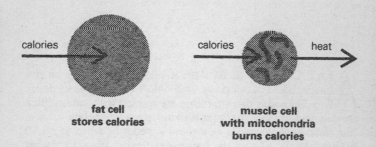

**fat cell
stores calories**

**muscle cell
with mitochondria
burns calories**

In summary, men have what it takes to lose weight through dieting and exercise: more fat-releasing lipolytic enzymes and more muscle. Women have what it takes to gain weight: more fat-storing enzymes and less muscle. The result is the stubborn female fat cell. It is concentrated in the hips and thighs, loves to store fat, hates to give up fat, and anxiously awaits the next diet. When I have shared this information with my clients, some have felt that they were doomed from the start. As one woman said, "Forget menstruation, this is the real Eve's curse." Well, curse or not, this is how a woman's body functions. You *must* accept that medical fact and work with your female physiology. Unfortunately, most women work against their physiology and turn to restrictive diets in desperation. Before you go to that extreme, please read the next chapter—because when you diet, your female fat cells fight back. And win.

■

Chapter Two

YOU CAN'T STARVE
A FAT CELL

A FAT CELL awakens with a smile. "This may be my lucky day. It's Monday, she didn't eat breakfast, drank two diet sodas this morning, ate a salad with lemon juice for lunch, and now she's fantasizing about chocolate eclairs. She must have started a new diet—spread the word to all 30 billion fat cells. Put up the barricades, recruit the extra forces . . . we must unite and thrive."

If fat cells could communicate (and sometimes it seems they can), this is a likely conversation they would have each time you start a new diet. No matter how hard you try to starve yourself, you cannot starve your fat cells. They won't let you. There is a built-in protective mechanism that ensures their survival.

To help you understand why it is impossible to starve a fat cell, let's take a giant step back in history to analyze the development of fat storage in the human body. I'm sure that you have heard of Darwin's "survival of the fittest" theory. The weak perished and the strong survived, passing on their survival traits and adapting to their environment over time. There are many animal examples of survival of the fittest: the giraffe's long neck to reach high foliage, the tree frog's skin color for camouflage, the skunk's scent to ward off enemies. When it comes to human adaptation, survival of the fittest may really be "survival of the fattest."

Thousands of years ago, periodic food shortages were a way

of life. They were the result of famine, drought, and catastrophe. Many died from starvation, but some people lived. Who were more likely to live? Those people with more body fat and bigger fat cells. They had more calories stored to withstand the food shortage. So, the fatter people lived and passed along their traits to the next generation. As "the fatter the better" trait was passed along from generation to generation, it became stronger and more specialized—and we became fatter beings.

Not only were there famines, but the famines were followed by feasting times. The body came to realize that the more efficiently it stored fat during feasting times, the fatter it would be and the more likely it would be to survive during a famine. The result of the famine/feast cycle on the development of our fat physiology is twofold:

1. Those people with *larger fat cells* survived the famine and passed along their trait.
2. Those people who were *more efficient fat storers* during feasting times survived the famine and passed along their trait.

We have inherited big, stubborn fat cells that love to store fat and hate to give it up.

So, throughout time, large and efficient fat cells have been linked to the survival of the human race. Hence, the survival of the fattest theory. And wouldn't you figure, this survival mechanism is stronger for women than for men. A man's body wants to protect itself for a couple of months of famine. A woman's body wants to protect itself for nine months of famine. Why nine months? You guessed it—what if a woman were pregnant when a famine hit? A woman's body not only wants to store fat to protect itself but also her developing child. Whether or not there is any remote chance of pregnancy, the fat cells prepare for the possibility. It's like an insurance policy for survival.

Based on this anthropological analysis, you could simply blame your weight problem on your ancestors and throw in the towel in defeat. But it is not that simple. What you do today has an even greater influence on your fat cells than what occurred thousands of years ago.

Your body may have learned the survival of the fattest lesson from your ancestors, but you keep giving it a refresher course on fat protection each time you go on a diet, and a refresher course on fat storage each time you go off a diet and back to your old eating habits. The famine/feast cycle of yesterday is the diet/binge cycle of today.

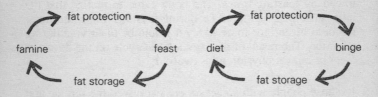

If you are the type of person who needs scientific, quantitative, factual, biochemical information to convince you that you can't starve a fat cell no matter how hard you try, read on and pay close attention. I'll relate everything to the physiology of the fat cell and the enzyme systems.

When you go on a diet, the red warning lights flash and the biochemical changes begin. First, there is the activation and multiplication of the fat-storing lipogenic enzymes. While you are on a diet, your body is actually trying to store more fat, but the real reason for the activation of the lipogenic enzymes is so that you will be better equipped to store plenty of fat after the diet. Research done at Cedars-Sinai Medical Center and other institutions has found that low-calorie diets at least double the lipogenic storage enzymes. *Women already have more storage enzymes than men, and dieting doubles them.*

Your fat cells are threatened and respond to the possible famine (your latest diet) by becoming at least twice as efficient at storage. The next time you go on a diet, your fat cells will be more likely to survive because they are larger, stronger, and more stubborn. Your fat cells are always thinking about your survival. Isn't that nice of them?

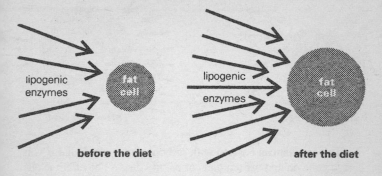

lipogenic enzymes — fat cell

before the diet

lipogenic enzymes — fat cell

after the diet

Of course, you lose some fat when you restrict calories and lose weight, but your fat cells become less efficient at losing fat. Your body wants to save its fat, not lose it. Again, it's a protective mechanism that ensures survival. Research has shown that dieting can reduce the fat-releasing lipolytic enzymes by 50 percent. *Women already have fewer releasing enzymes than men, and dieting cuts them in half.*

So there you have it. The survival of the fattest theory affects the fat-enzyme system. You become twice as efficient in storage and enlarging your fat cells, and half as efficient in releasing and shrinking your fat cells.

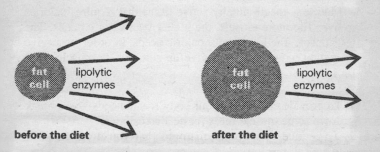

fat cell — lipolytic enzymes

before the diet

fat cell — lipolytic enzymes

after the diet

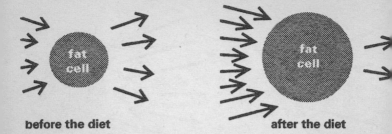

before the diet   **after the diet**

This is what can happen with just one diet cycle. What if you nave gone on and off ten diets or twenty diets? The effect is cumulative. You have even more storage enzymes and fewer releasing enzymes with each diet cycle. Have you ever wondered why each time you go on a diet, you lose the weight more slowly and gain the weight back more quickly? I hope that this helps you to understand why. With each diet you are starting with fewer fat-releasing lipolytic enzymes and more fat-storing lipogenic enzymes. With each diet you have less of what it takes to lose weight and more of what it takes to gain weight.

Wait! the bad news about dieting isn't over yet. Not only do your fat cells become bigger and stronger, but your mus-:le cells become smaller and weaker. Your muscle cells do not have the protective bodyguards that your fat cells do. *Fat cells won't starve, but muscle cells will.*

Muscle is metabolically active tissue that requires calories :o live. The more muscle, the higher your caloric needs. The less muscle, the lower your caloric needs. In order to survive starvation, your body will give up some of its muscle mass for two reasons:

1. To provide energy for your body's vital needs—you break down some muscle mass for needed calories.
2. To reduce your metabolism so that you don't need as many calories to live.

YOU CAN'T STARVE A FAT CELL

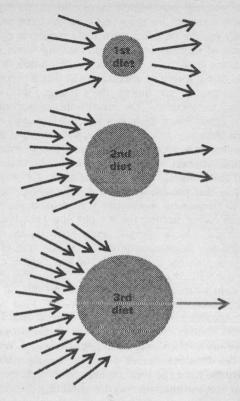

(The number of arrows in this, and in all diagrams in this book, do not reflect the number of enzymes; they are to help you visualize the storage and release of fat.)

When you go on a diet, your body actually wants to get rid of some of its muscle to reduce your metabolism and conserve energy. Some of the weight that you lose is muscle weight. This is not good. It may sound good, but it is not. The less muscle you have, the slower your metabolism, the less you can eat, and the less weight you will lose. Muscle burns calories; fat stores calories. The less you burn, the more you store, the more you weigh.

So, when you are on a diet, your body conserves calories by losing some of its muscle mass and burning fewer calories. When a calorie goes to the muscle cell to be burned, the muscle cell knows that it might be sacrificed and that it needs to conserve. "I'd better not burn this up; she's dieting. I'd better give it to the fat cell to conserve." You practice this conservation strategy all the time. When there is a gas shortage, you conserve fuel. When there is a money shortage, you conserve spending. And when there is a calorie shortage, you conserve energy.

Each time you go on a diet, you enter the conservation mode and lose muscle. You also lose some fat—but what's important is that the fat loss is not permanent; the muscle loss may be permanent. Each time you go off a diet and back to your old eating habits, the weight you gain back is not muscle weight, it's fat weight. Your fat cells are equipped with double the storage enzymes to quickly and efficiently gain fat. It is possible to replenish the lost muscle mass, but only exercise will do it.

"Why didn't someone warn me about all this fat survival physiology before I went on my first diet?" Tina began the dieting game about six years ago. "I thought that I was fat then at 150 pounds, but look at me now at 186 pounds. I would give my soul to weigh 150 pounds again." When Tina went on her first restrictive diet, she weighed about 150 pounds. By the time she went on her fourth diet, the result of the weight loss/weight gain was devastating.

	Pre-Diet	First Diet Cycle	Second Diet Cycle	Third Diet Cycle	Fourth Diet Cycle
Total weight	150	156	164	175	186
Muscle weight	108	104	99	96	92
Fat weight	42	52	65	79	94

Each diet cycle is the result of weight loss (muscle and fat) while she was on the diet, and weight gain (fat only) when she went off the diet. By her fourth diet cycle, Tina had lost sixteen pounds of muscle and gained fifty-two pounds of fat. It's no wonder that Tina and many others claim that they gain weight just by thinking about food. They have been on many diets, have lost muscle, gained fat, and have slowed down their metabolisms. Their bodies need fewer calories and are more efficient at storing those fewer calories as fat.

Maybe it is time to define the word "diet." The real meaning of diet is what you eat on a daily basis, but society has changed that to mean a restriction of calories. Whenever you restrict calories below the level that your body needs to function, your body senses starvation and switches into the conservation mode. The more you restrict calories and the longer you diet, the more muscle you will lose and the more your fat cells will fight back. An 800-calorie diet will do more damage than a 1,200-calorie diet. A two-month diet will do more damage than a two-week diet. But even the Monday through Thursday dieters will see the negative effects of their fat, muscle, and metabolism over time. It takes only seventy-two hours of restriction for your fat cells to begin protection and your muscle cells to begin sacrifice.

I thought about not sharing this last bit of the survival of the fattest theory with you, but it may be what it takes for you to give up dieting forever.

Sit down and secure yourself. Diets not only make your fat cells bigger, they may also make your fat cells multiply. Forget the old fat-cell theory that you increase the number of fat cells in your body only during infancy, early childhood, and adolescence (for women only). The latest shocking discovery is that fat cells can divide at any age—and dieting may help. As we have discussed, with dieting the body learns a lesson and is always preparing for the next diet. The *larger the fat cell*, the more likely it is that you will survive the next diet. And—the *more fat cells* you have, the more you can store, and the more likely it is that you will survive the next diet. Once your fat cells are filled up to their maximum size, they may divide so that they can store even more fat in anticipation of your next diet. If you were on a diet right now, you might be giving birth to a new thigh fat cell at this very moment. I know it is a horrible thought—but you are not on a diet, so you are preventing the birth of a new fat cell.

The bottom line is: If you want to gain weight, go on and off diets for the rest of your life. Dieting does such a good job of helping you gain weight that one of the newest methods of enabling underweight people to gain weight is to put them on and off short dieting cycles.

If you want to store more fat . . .
If you want larger fat cells . . .
If you want more fat cells . . .
If you want less muscle mass . . .
If you want a slower metabolism . . .
If you want to gain weight . . .
. . . GO ON A DIET

And if you want to be at a greater risk for disease, go on a diet. I realize that most women diet for appearance and not for health reasons, but if you are health-conscious, listen to this: You would be healthier staying moderately overweight than losing your excess weight and gaining it back. If you were ten pounds overweight, lost the ten pounds on a diet, then regained the ten pounds after the diet, you would be at a significant higher risk for heart disease, cancer, and diabetes than if you just stayed ten pounds overweight. With dieting, even though your weight may not change, your body composition does, and you are fatter after the diet than before the diet. It's not your weight but the fat on your body that increases disease risk.

In moments of frustration, low self-esteem, and desperation, you may start thinking about dieting again. You may have a friend who just lost thirty-five pounds on the latest diet craze and looks terrific. You may have a special occasion coming up and want to look your best, which in your mind is a size 10. You may have read about a new diet that promises a 95 percent success rate. Diets are tempting because they make persuasive promises of quick results, but those results are temporary. Don't believe the success rates of diets; instead, use the information in this chapter to read between the lines.

If this is the claim: "This diet guarantees a twenty-pound weight loss in one month or your money back," read between the lines and you will see that it really means: "This (restrictive, unsatisfying) diet guarantees a twenty-pound (seven of it from muscle) weight loss (and a slower metabolism) in one month (and a twelve-pound fat gain over the next month) or your money back."

Who in their right mind would be tempted by this diet? Hopefully, not you after you have read this chapter. If you ever get the urge to diet, please read this chapter again, and again, and again. Memorize the phrase, *"You can't starve a fat cell."*

"I am completely depressed. In the first chapter you told me that because I am a woman, I have big, stubborn fat cells. Now you are telling me that dieting makes them even bigger and more stubborn. I am a *woman* who has been a *professional dieter* all her life. Is there any hope for me?" That's the very purpose of this book—and yes, there is hope. The OFF Plan will work with your female physiology, undo the damage of dieting, and help you stay off dieting forever.

.. You can't compare apples and pears—women must be treated differently with regard to weight loss.
2. You can't starve a fat cell—there is a built-in protective mechanism that won't let you.

Then, what *can* you do to permanently lose weight and outsmart your female fat cells? You can follow the OFF Plan. The good news is that your exercise habits, and food choices can either fuel a female fat cell or fool it. The choice is yours.

Chapter Three

■

THE **OFF** PLAN:
6 STRATEGIES TO
OUTSMART **F**EMALE **F**AT

W HEN ONE of my clients, Jill, called and woke me up one night at eleven-thirty with something that could not wait, I knew it had to be important. She had run into an old college friend that night who raved about how great Jill looked and asked her what new diet she was on. Jill laughed and responded that she had given up diets about a year ago. Her friend was about to start a rumor that Jill had undergone liposuction from head to toe when Jill finally told her, "I've simply switched my female fat cells off with the **OFF** Plan."

You, too, will switch your fat cells off with the diet-free, medically sound, lifestyle approach of the **OFF** Plan to:

OUTSMART
FEMAL
FAT

Through a series of 6 logical and realistic strategies that focus on how you eat, not what you eat, your female fat cells will be tricked into switching off. You have been "feeding" your fat cells for most of your life through dieting and overeating. The **OFF** Plan strategies feed your body, not your fat cells.

In order for you to fully understand exactly how the **OFF** Plan switches your fat cells off, I first need to discuss what switches them on. You already know about the effects of estrogen, but let me summarize so that you can view the whole picture. The surge of estrogen during puberty flipped the switch on, and the fat cells of the hips, buttocks, and thighs were awakened. Then, for many women, they are given some extra voltage with oral contraceptives, pregnancy, and estrogen replacement.

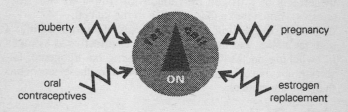

When I shared this information with my husband, he commented, "It sounds like women are power plants for fat production. Too bad you can't just call the electric company and tell them to cut the power." The situation is not that extreme, but, compared to a man's, a woman's fat cell does have more power for storage. I have used this analogy of a light switch turning the fat storage power on and off to help you visualize

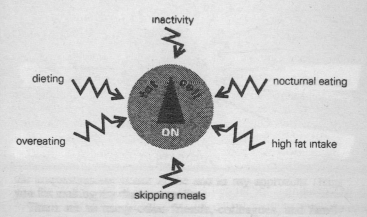

the factors influencing your fat cells. It is certainly not as easy as flipping a switch, but the "light switch" analogy will give you an awareness of what activates your fat cells and what deactivates them.

So, simply being a woman is enough to switch your fat cells on. Unfortunately, you do not have much control over the effects of estrogen on female fat. But there are other choices women make that give life to the fat cell.

Dieting, overeating, skipping meals, nocturnal eating, a high fat intake, and inactivity are just as effective as estrogen in switching on the fat cell by activating the lipogenic, fat-storing enzymes. But, on the positive side, these are habits that you can control.

DIETING

As discussed in Chapter 2, *dieting is the fat cell's best friend.* Fat cells have an excellent memory. As soon as you go on another diet, your fat cells realize "here she goes again" and know exactly what to do. They are threatened and don't want to starve, so they switch on the storage power for survival with the lipogenic enzymes.

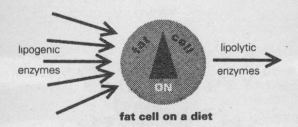

lipogenic
enzymes

lipolytic
enzymes

fat cell on a diet

OVEREATING

Overeating is the fat cell's second best friend. Whenever you eat more calories than your body needs at a given time, the lipogenic enzymes are called upon to store the excess in your fat cells. Fat is the storage form of energy. If your body needs 500 calories to function at noon today, but you eat 1,000 calories, that excess 500 calories (no matter where it is coming from: pasta, fruit, or cookies) will be converted to and stored as fat.

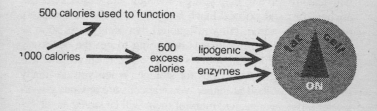

Both dieting and overeating switch the fat cell on—they are partners in crime. They work in tandem to create an endless cycle of feeling out of control. There is no in-between—you're either dieting or binging.

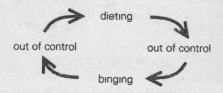

What day do you usually start a diet? Silly question—it's always Monday. Would you ever start a diet on Friday night? You need the weekend to vacuum out the cupboards and refrigerator in preparation for Monday's deprivation. What kind of meal do you eat to celebrate the end of your diet? You get the idea—with this dieting/binging cycle, it's no wonder that women gain weight. Their fat cells are constantly in the storage mode.

SKIPPING MEALS

Skipping a meal is like going on a mini-diet. Fat cells have calorie radars. When you skip a meal, you may think, "That's 500 calories that won't get me," but your body is deprived of calories for hours and the fat cells switch on. This deprivation in calories will actually serve to help you gain weight. For example, if you ate breakfast and skipped lunch today, your body was probably hungry at noontime, but you ignored that hunger. As soon as your body realized that it was not going to get the necessary nourishment to function, it did what it needed to survive by activating the lipogenic enzymes for storage. When you do finally give your body food at dinner, your fat cells are anxiously waiting for those calories, and more of them will be stored as fat. By skipping a meal you fool only yourself, not your fat cells.

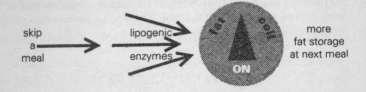

NOCTURNAL EATING

Eating at night feeds the fat cell because your metabolism and caloric needs are lowest at night. The majority of us eat our largest meal at dinner and many top it off with snacking while watching TV. These are excess calories that our bodies do not need. The fact that 55 percent of the evening TV commercials are for food may send us wandering into the kitchen with "snack amnesia." As Virginia describes it, a commercial comes on for potato chips and she doesn't even realize that she has gotten up from the couch, grabbed the chips from the cupboard, sat back down, and devoured them—until the en-

---

tire bag is empty. Most of the food you eat at night is not for your body, it's for your fat cells.

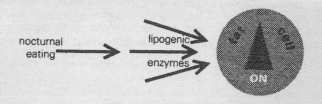

✕ HIGH FAT INTAKE

A high fat intake and a large fat cell go hand in hand. Fat cells love fat and are undoubtedly more efficient at storing fat than at storing starch and protein. <u>The more fat in your diet, the more likely it will become fat in your fat cell.</u> It makes sense if we spend a moment thinking about it. If you eat a loaf of French bread, your body will use some of it (maybe one-third of the loaf) to function. The remaining two-thirds of the loaf needs to be converted to fat before it can be stored as fat in your fat cell. If you eat a stick of butter (yuck!), it doesn't need to be converted, it already is fat and more easily slips into a fat cell.

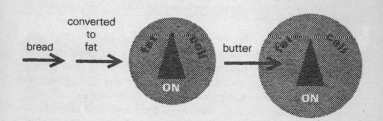

INACTIVITY

Finally, and perhaps most importantly, inactivity keeps the fat cell eternally happy. <u>Without exercise, there are few fat-releas-</u>

ing lipolytic enzymes to compete with the fat-storing lipogenic enzymes. The fat cells stay full and content. Until now, we have discussed only what activates and multiplies the lipogenic enzymes for storage. The *only* factor that influences the lipolytic enzymes for release of fat is regular physical activity. A sedentary person's fat cell lacks the machinery to make the fat cell smaller—its lipolytic enzymes are in hibernation. An active person's fat cell has lipolytic enzymes working around the clock.

 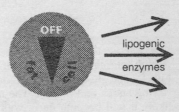

lipogenic
enzymes

sedentary fat cell   **physically active fat cell**

Now that you know everything about a fat cell and how to turn your female fat cells on and gain weight, how do you switch your fat cells off and lose weight?

THE OFF PLAN

The **OFF** Plan consists of 6 effective strategies that switch your fat cells off because they are directly opposed to what switches your fat cells on. For example, if nocturnal eating activates the lipogenic enzymes, then daytime eating deactivates the lipogenic enzymes and prevents fat storage. If inactivity limits the lipolytic enzymes, then exercise stimulates the lipolytic enzymes to release fat.

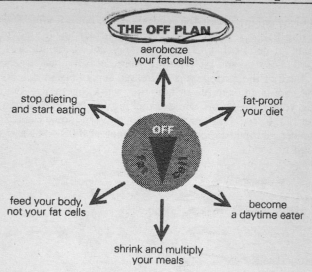

THE OFF PLAN

aerobicize
your fat cells

stop dieting
and start eating

fat-proof
your diet

OFF

feed your body,
not your fat cells

become
a daytime eater

shrink and multiply
your meals

Switching Fat Cells ON	Switching Fat Cells OFF
Inactivity	Aerobicize your fat cells
Dieting	Stop dieting and start eating
Overeating	Feed your body, not your fat cells
Skipping meals	Shrink and multiply your meals
Nocturnal eating	Become a daytime eater
High fat intake	Fat-proof your diet

As I will discuss throughout this program, regular aerobic exercise is by far the top strategy. If you do nothing else, exercise! But to permanently and successfully outsmart your female fat cells, regular aerobic exercise *and* the OFF Plan eating strategies is the winning combination for making your fat cells smaller. Exercise will ensure fat release, and eating habit changes will prevent fat storage. To most of my clients' surprise, the <u>OFF</u> strategies do not emphasize what to eat and what not to eat. <u>What you eat does not trigger your fat cells as much as why, when, and how much you eat.</u> Your food choices are important for general health, but it's your overall eating habits that have the greatest influence on switching your fat cells off. Only one strategy out of six focuses on food choices—and fat-proofing your diet is the last strategy!

Each of the strategies is addressed separately in this book, but here is an example of how they work together in switching your fat cells off. Before making the **OFF** Plan a part of her life, Chrisi didn't exercise, dieted every January and September, skipped lunch, overate dinner at 8:00 P.M., and ate high-fat foods.

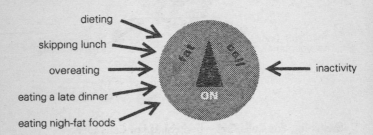

After following the **OFF** Plan for about nine months, she went on a sailing trip with some friends. Her friends could not believe that she ate the way she did, looked great, and maintained her weight during the trip while they all gained weight. They commented that it seemed as if she was eating all day long and eating whatever she wanted to. In reality, the **OFF** Plan gave her the freedom to eat like a naturally thin person—she didn't deny herself, ate when she was hungry, ate small frequent meals so that she was seldom overeating, and didn't eat late at night (well, except for one 9:00 P.M. dinner). She also kept up with her exercise program. She enjoyed the trip and outsmarted her fat cells at the same time.

So there's the scientific basis of the **OFF** Plan and the explanation of how it works to switch your fat cells off. *The end result is that you will change the enzyme system of your* *fat cells. You will have more releasing enzymes than storage enzymes—and that's the only way to permanently shrink your fat cells.* I hope that you are encouraged by the **OFF** Plan and eager to begin practicing the strategies. But before you dive in, I want to prepare you for a successful program by enhancing your readiness, commitment, and motivation. They are your initial ingredients for success.

■

Chapter Four

ARE YOU READY FOR THE <u>OFF</u> PLAN?

ARE YOU ready to get started with the <u>OFF</u> Plan? You may be thinking, "I'm not sure" or, "Maybe I'll be ready next month" or, "I'll never be ready." Remember, you are *not* getting ready to start a new diet. Diets are difficult to follow, and before you begin, you have to psyche yourself up for a month of restrictions, isolation, and deprivation. I'm not asking you to prepare for deprivation. I'm asking you to prepare for a new, natural way of eating—for the next three months, the next year, the next ten years, the rest of your life.

Some of my clients ask, "Why bother preparing? Why can't I just do it?" Because preparation ensures success. Would you ever take a test without preparing for it? Would you ever go into an interview without preparing for it? If you didn't prepare, you would most likely flunk the test and fail to get the job. As with anything you do in your life, lifestyle changes require preparation, commitment, and a plan of action. Think of other lifestyle changes that you have made: education, marriage, career, relocation—they all required preparation.

To be successful in outsmarting your female fat cells, you must prepare yourself psychologically for the <u>OFF</u> Plan:

- You must believe in it.
- You must share the <u>OFF</u> philosophies.

- You must have a full understanding of your female fat cells.
- You must replace your diet mentality with a lifestyle mentality.
- You must think in terms of permanent, not temporary, weight loss.
- You must think in terms of slow, not fast, weight loss.
- You must think in terms of fat loss, not weight loss.
- You must have realistic goals that are attainable.

The first step is to get ready, prepare yourself, and provide a framework for success. This first step forward may be the most difficult because it means commitment. You've already made some commitment by purchasing this book, reading the first three chapters, and gaining knowledge of the female fat cell—how it differs from a male fat cell and what activates it. Nevertheless, *commitment* can be a frightening word.

What scared Joanne was that she was committing herself to a program that would last the rest of her life: "The only thing that I have ever committed to for the rest of my life was brushing my teeth after every meal."

But where did that lifelong commitment come from? First, Joanne was constantly reminded by her parents to brush her teeth. Then, goals were set for her to do it on a daily basis. She received the positive reinforcement to continue brushing her teeth because of the benefit of better dental health and fewer cavities. Her commitment and lifetime behavior developed over time in a systematic way. That's how behavior change works. It may not be as simple as brushing your teeth, and your parents probably won't remind you to exercise or to eat when you are hungry—but it is a series of small steps that naturally leads to a new behavior.

Like Joanne, you will be relieved to hear that although the end result is lifelong change, the OFF Plan is a series of small, step-by-step changes that are slowly integrated over the next three months. By setting and achieving short-term goals, the progressive changes will eventually become permanent changes. Joanne was not willing to commit to exercise for the rest of her life, but she was willing to start by setting realistic goals every two weeks and committing to scheduling exercise into her life. I know this is hard to believe, but at the end of three months, she actually wanted to continue exercising.

That's the way the OFF Plan works. The small, progressive changes over the first three months make you feel better and provide the motivation and commitment for the rest of your life. Eventually, the new behaviors replace the old ones, and the new, learned behaviors become effortless. The changes you make are so natural and realistic that you don't have to think about them anymore. You wake up one day realizing that you are exercising every Monday, Wednesday, and Friday. You are automatically ordering your sandwiches without mayonnaise. You are not even considering seconds. Rocky road ice cream doesn't enter your mind even when you are stressed. Doesn't this positive, natural, and healthy approach make much more sense than "yo-yo" dieting? Dieting is negative, unnatural, and unhealthy—and does not change behaviors. The OFF Plan does.

So, are you ready for the OFF Plan? The three questionnaires in this chapter will assess your level of readiness, enhance your awareness, and identify the attitude changes necessary to fully prepare you for a successful 3-month program. Without changing attitudes and beliefs, you cannot change behaviors. Without changing behaviors, you cannot change your body.

Do You Need to Psychologically Prepare Yourself for the OFF Plan?

No doubt your feelings about your weight and your body have been influenced by society's pressure for thinness and by the diet industry. Fill in this questionnaire to discover the effects of this influence on your feelings, attitudes, and behaviors.

	YES	NO
1. I weigh myself daily.	—	—
2. My weight determines how I feel about myself.	—	—
3. When I discover I've gained a pound, I panic.	—	—
4. I want to lose weight quickly.	—	—
5. My weight prevents me from achieving other goals in my life.	—	—
6. I want to lose weight for my husband/significant other.	—	—
7. I want to lose weight for an upcoming event.	—	—
8. I want to achieve the "ideal" body.	—	—
9. I avoid mirrors and window reflections.	—	—
10. I'm depressed when I look through fashion magazines.	—	—
11. I avoid social events because of my weight.		
12. I dislike my body.	—	—

The greater the number of statements you answered "yes," the more you need to deprogram the "diet mentality" and society's influence—the more you need to focus on psychologically preparing yourself for successful lifestyle change. In my experience, most women answer yes to 50 percent to 100 percent of the statements, so if you did, you are not alone. Society's pressure for thinness and the ideal body has given most women a negative body image and the diet mentality.

Before you can begin making changes in your habits, you must first make some changes in your attitudes and how you feel about yourself.

You must be ready to disregard the scale. The scale does not tell you how much muscle and fat you have; it only tells you how much your whole body weighs—muscle, fat, bones, and organs. It is impossible to evaluate how much fat you have lost and how much muscle you have gained. The scale can also sabotage your efforts. If you discover you have gained a couple of pounds, you are depressed and eat. If you discover that you have lost a couple of pounds, you rejoice and eat to reward yourself. Any way you look at it, the numbers on the scale can make you eat.

I don't even have a scale in my office. When clients come in for their first appointment, they quickly scan the room and ask, "Ok, where's the scale? In the closet?" When I tell them that I don't have one, they are surprised and sometimes a little perturbed: "You mean I fasted all day yesterday for nothing?" That's what the scale does to you. Do yourself a favor and throw away the scale or put it in the garage—at least for the next three months. Don't let the numbers on the scale determine how you feel about yourself.

If you find that you can't part with the scale, do not weigh yourself more than once a week and develop more of an intellectual rather than an emotional relationship with your scale. Keep in mind:

- Weight can fluctuate as much as five pounds a day because of normal fluctuations in your body's water balance.
- If you are premenstrual or recently had a high-salt meal, increased weight may be water weight.
- Your weight on the scale gives you no indication of your fat mass and muscle mass.
- Muscle weighs more than fat. If you are exercising and gain two pounds of muscle and lose two pounds of fat— the scale won't budge, but your body has.
- Notice how your clothes fit and how you look in the mirror.

You must be ready to lose weight slowly. If you want to lose weight quickly, this plan is not for you. A traditional weight-loss diet may promise rapid weight loss, but it will also ensure rapid weight gain. If you want to lose weight permanently, then prepare yourself for natural, slow changes in your eating habits and your body. You may have heard that "losing one to two pounds a week is a safe weight loss." "Safe" means that you will probably not harm your health. "Safe" does not mean permanent—*slow* means permanent.

You must determine if weight is serving a special purpose in your life. For some women, their weight is a useful tool to prevent them from achieving goals. After struggling with her weight for nine years, Barbara finally came to the conclusion that her weight made life easy and nonthreatening. As long as she was overweight, she felt that she didn't have to develop other areas of her life such as career, family, and education. Her weight was an excuse for not experiencing life's successes and failures. As soon as Barbara acknowledged and dealt with these issues, she didn't need her weight anymore and was able to lose weight with the OFF Plan.

Does excess weight serve a purpose in your life? For some of my clients, excess weight made them feel powerful, strong, and was a means of self-defense. For others, it was a barrier to prevent relationships and intimacy. If your excess weight is serving a certain purpose and perceived need in your life, you'll carry your weight until you don't need it anymore.

You must want to lose weight for yourself—not your husband, partner, mother, doctor, or girlfriends. When you lose weight for someone else, it is almost never permanent. Often, the goal to lose weight is in combination with an upcoming special event—a wedding, a class reunion, a vacation. You are not losing weight for you; you are losing weight for the event. When the event is over, your commitment is over, and your weight gain begins. Sue lost twenty-two pounds for a trip to Hawaii. She regained ten pounds while on the trip and the remaining twelve pounds within her first month back. Sound familiar? Lose weight for *you* and become internally motivated, not externally motivated by others or an event. *Why do you want to lose weight?*

You must find your own "ideal body," one that is realistic and attainable. If you live in a Western society, it is almost impossible not to be influenced by society's ideal figure. The messages are loud and clear: Thin is beautiful, and if you are not thin, then you are inferior, unsuccessful, and an outcast. The quest for thinness is a product of the twentieth century—

really of the last thirty years or so. The acceptable natural womanly figure used to have curves and hips. Sizes 2, 4, and 6 didn't even exist. Today, if you are bigger than a size 14, *you* don't exist (at least in department stores).

So what happened thirty years ago? We could blame it on Twiggy, but there was a drastic shift in the entire fashion industry. As the ideal body has gotten thinner, the average American woman has gotten fatter. It is no wonder that most women have a negative body image and dislike their bodies. No matter how hard we diet, we can't look like a Madison Avenue model. The average model is five feet ten and a half inches tall and weighs 114 pounds. The average woman is five feet four inches tall and weighs 140 pounds—and hasn't seen 114 pounds this side of puberty. For over 90 percent of us, the ideal body simply is not biologically possible. And that small percentage for which it is possible, well, they are probably models.

Now society is putting additional pressure on women. The latest ideal figure is still thin—but with muscles and large breasts. Help! Nothing short of plastic surgery and spending three hours a day lifting weights can accomplish that feat. Haven't we had enough? Let's let the fashion industry sell us the latest styles, not the ideal body.

Your personal "ideal body" is not determined by the media, the woman next door, or the weight charts. You have your own optimal weight that is influenced by genetics, body structure, pregnancy, and age. Your ideal body is not what you weighed at age twenty, even though you may have been told that this is a realistic goal. As you grow older, metabolism slows down and body shape changes. Pregnancy and menopause can also permanently change the shape of your body.

Your personal, optimal weight takes all of these factors into consideration. Optimal weight is the weight at which you feel the most comfortable, energetic, and healthy, a weight that can be maintained without your having to eat like a rabbit. Think about your weight goal:

• Is it realistic?
• Does it take into consideration genetics and age?

- Does it take into consideration pregnancy?
- Have you ever been at this weight before? If so, have you been able to maintain it naturally and without starvation?

If your weight goal and desired "ideal body" is unrealistic, you'll never be successful. Reassess your weight goals. Better yet, replace your weight goals with body fat goals. More about that at the end of this chapter.

You must feel good about yourself and your body now.
You must be prepared to accept your body and learn to like it. If you have "saddlebags that could ride the Pony Express" now, you'll always have some saddlebags. If you are broad-chested now, you'll have a broad chest after weight loss.

If you dislike your body because it is not "perfect," self-starvation is not the answer. A negative body image usually does not improve with weight loss. Many women find that achieving the "ideal" body does not make them happy; they still dislike their thighs, their jobs, and their lives. "Ideal body" and "happy life" are not necessarily synonymous.

What do you like about your body? When I ask my clients this question, nine out of ten say either "absolutely nothing" or "my eyelashes." To help them accept and respect their bodies, I have them analyze each part of their bodies to find something that they like about each part. They are pleasantly surprised to discover that they do like some aspects of their bodies, and they feel better about themselves. Would you like to give this activity a try? Analyze each of the following body parts and search for something you like in each area. For example, you may like the size of your feet, the calf muscles of your legs, or the birthmark on your back. "Nothing" is not an acceptable answer.

Your feet:	_____
Your legs:	_____
Your trunk:	_____
Your arms:	_____
Your hands:	_____
Your head:	_____

By filling out the Do You Need to Psychologically Prepare Yourself for the **OFF** Plan? questionnaire and becoming
more aware of your attitudes, your feelings, and your reasons
for weight loss, you have begun to mentally prepare yourself
to begin making small, realistic changes. You have begun to
give up the "diet mentality" and accept the "lifestyle mentality." If you feel that you need further assistance, get some
help from family, friends, or a counselor.

What Are Your Female Factors?

The message from society may be that thin is good, but the
message from your physiology is that fat is better—and your
physiology is a lot more powerful than society. You may not
be able to control the fact that you are a woman with estrogen and extra body fat, but it is important for you to become
aware of all the effects of estrogen on your fat cells, what we
will call the "female factors."

	YES	NO
Do you menstruate?	——	——
Are you pear-shaped?	——	——
Are you currently taking oral contraceptives?	——	——
Have you taken oral contraceptives in the past?	——	——
Have you been pregnant within the past year?	——	——
Have you ever been pregnant?	——	——
Have you been pregnant two or more times?	——	——
Have you entered menopause?	——	——
Are you on estrogen replacement?	——	——
Is/was your mother overweight?	——	——
If you have sisters, are they (she) overweight?	——	——

The greater number of questions you answered "yes," the
more female factors you have and the more stubborn your fat
cells may be. I wish there was enough research to give you
some idea of the strength of these factors—that if you had
five yesses, it would take you six months; of if you answered

eight yesses, it would take you nine months. What I *can* tell you is that the greater number of female factors you have, the longer it will take. Don't despair—*it means that the* OFF *Plan was designed specifically for you.* Chapter 13 will discuss some of these female factors in more depth, but I'll give you a brief explanation now for some understanding.

Menstruation means that you are experiencing normal hormonal fluctuations each month. Being a menstruating woman is enough to activate the fat cells in your buttocks, hips, and thighs. Research has shown that the more **pear-shaped** you are, the more sensitive your fat cells are to the effects of estrogen, and the more fat-storing enzymes you have.

If you are using **oral contraceptives,** the extra estrogen in your system may increase body fat from 1 percent to 3 percent. If you have used oral contraceptives in the past, the influence will not be as strong today, but your fat cells may still be slightly bigger from taking the Pill five years ago. Fat cells have an amazing memory.

If you have recently been **pregnant,** the high estrogen levels for nine months created a fat frenzy. Increased body fat is necessary for a healthy pregnancy, but trying to lose that last ten pounds is extremely difficult for most women. The more times you have been pregnant, the more body fat you have stored, particularly in the hips, buttocks, and thighs.

If you are **menopausal** or postmenopausal, estrogen levels may be lower, but your metabolism takes a nose dive and weight gain is common. Because of lower estrogen levels, that weight gain accumulates in the abdominal area—and a woman's fat distribution begins to resemble a man's. If you are a menopausal woman on **estrogen replacement therapy,** the fat cells of the buttocks, hips, and thighs are activated again. As one client said, "Now I have fat everywhere!"

If your **mother** and/or **sisters** are overweight, then you may have a genetic tendency to be overweight as well. There is a great debate over genetics versus environment: Are you overweight because of your mother's genes or because you grew up in an overweight family environment that was sedentary and food-focused? It's probably a combination of both factors.

The solution is not to forgo oral contraceptives, avoid pregnancy, discontinue estrogen replacement therapy, and surgically remove your overweight genes (sorry, there is no such surgery). These are necessary parts of being a woman. *The solution is to acknowledge all of your female factors, to use them to set realistic goals, and to put an even greater commitment into the* OFF *Plan—because it was designed especially for you.*

Now for some good news: There are some definite benefits to these female factors. First of all, a certain amount of body fat is essential to being a woman—for maintaining healthy menstruation and childbearing. When a woman's body fat drops too far (below 18 percent), she loses her femininity: menstrual periods cease or become irregular, breasts become smaller, and infertility can result.

Second, we have longevity on our side. Women live about eight years longer than men. Maybe we should keep our longevity secrets to ourselves, but estrogen and the pear-shaped body have been strongly associated with a lower rate of heart disease, diabetes, and certain cancers. Men may have less fat, but they are apple-shaped and have more disease. I don't know about you, but I'll take a little extra hip fat over disease any day.

What Are Your Fat Statistics?

One more area of preparation before you get started—your fat statistics. To measure changes and your success in the program, you need to know the amount of fat on your body today and where it is deposited. The key word here is *fat*. I really don't care how much you weigh; I do care about how fat you are.

BODY COMPOSITION ANALYSIS: **DATE:** _____
   WEIGHT: ____
   % BODY FAT: ____
   POUNDS OF FAT: ____
   POUNDS OF MUSCLE: ____

BODY MEASUREMENTS: **DATE:** _____
    BREAST INCHES: ___
    WAIST INCHES: ___
    HIP INCHES·   ___
    THIGH INCHES·   ___

As we discussed in the introduction, the "real" weight loss is pounds of fat lost, not pounds of weight lost. It is also beneficial to gain weight, as long as it is muscle weight. The only way to determine your fat and muscle mass is to have your body composition analyzed. There are a number of methods available, but the following two are the most accurate.

1 *Underwater weighing.* This method is based on the concept that fat floats and muscle sinks in water. If your body has a lot of fat, you will float more and therefore weigh less in water. If you are lean and muscular, you'll sink more and therefore weigh more in water. It's a positive sign when you weigh a lot with this method.
2. *Skinfold measurements.* This method is based on the "if you can pinch more than an inch, you're overweight" concept. An instrument pinches the fat on your arm, hip, and thigh (and sometimes other areas) and measures its thickness to determine the amount of fat in your body.

I realize that neither of these methods sounds like much fun. As one of my clients commented, "My choices are to get dunked in water or pinched!" They are not at all painful, and all of my clients have benefited from the experience because it has freed them from the scale. Once they realize the detailed information that body composition analysis gives them, they don't want to get on the scale ever again.

Cynthia was finally convinced to disregard the scale after her experience with the initial 3-month program. She had made great strides in changing her eating habits and was exercising four times a week. Even though she felt smaller and her clothes were looser, she was frustrated because the scale showed that she'd gained one pound. She was ready to bury the OFF Plan with her more than twenty previous diet failures when I convinced her to have her body composition tested again:

	Baseline	After 3 months	Change
Total Weight	138 lbs	139 lbs	+ 1 lb
% Body Fat	28 %	25 %	-3 %
Fat Weight	39 lbs	35 lbs	-4 lbs
Muscle Weight	99 lbs	104 lbs	+5 lbs

This gave her the motivating information that the scale couldn't. She discovered that she had really lost 3 percent body fat and four pounds of fat. She realized that the scale went up a pound because her exercise program resulted in a five-pound gain of muscle. To this day, Cynthia is "hooked" on body composition analysis.

Because of this detailed information that only body composition analysis can offer, I strongly encourage you to make it a part of your program. Still, some women are reluctant to have their body composition analyzed because they don't want to find out how fat they are. All you want is a baseline so you will be able to measure positive changes later. Where you are now isn't important; what you lose in the next three months is important. Whether you are 30 percent, 40 percent or 50 percent body fat, don't worry about it. You will see that percentage decrease and eventually get down to around 25 percent. Why 25 percent? Because if you are more than 25 percent body fat, you are increasing your risk of disease. If you want to get below 25 percent body fat, that's your own personal decision. But for general health and fitness, around 25 percent body fat is just fine.

When you decide to have your body composition analyzed, whatever method you choose (underwater weighing or skinfold measurements), I recommend that you be consistent. If you use underwater weighing for the initial measurements stick with it for future measurements. Switching from one method to another may not produce accurate numbers for measuring change.

The method you choose does, however, influence cost. The estimated cost ranges from $10 for skinfold measurements to about $30 for underwater weighing. If you are not aware of the availability of body composition analysis in your area, contact: registered dietitians, exercise physiologists, cardiologists, physicians' offices, health clubs, YWCAs and YMCAs, hospitals, or colleges and universities.

If you do not have your body composition analyzed, it is essential that you focus more on changes in body size than body weight: notice how you look in the mirror, how your clothes fit, and take measurements of your waist, hips, breasts, and thighs. Weight loss may be insignificant while body size changes are very significant because of a gain in muscle mass.

I'll say it one more time: Please throw away your scale, forget about your weight, focus on measuring changes in your body, and have your body composition analyzed. You'll be a happier person, you'll acknowledge real changes in your body, and you'll know a lot more about your level of fitness and health.

I hope that by having completed the three questionnaires in this chapter, you feel better prepared for the <u>OFF</u> Plan. You have gained an awareness of your attitudes, your body image, and your motivation. You have acknowledged the effects of estrogen on your body. You have (I hope) had your body composition analyzed, determined your fat statistics, and reassessed your goals.

Now, are you ready to get started with the <u>OFF</u> Plan? Not only do I want you to be successful in outsmarting your female fat cells, but I also want you to enjoy the steps to a leaner body and healthier lifestyle:

- Keep a sense of humor.
- Make the commitment.
- Throw away your scale.

- Lose weight for yourself.
- Have the patience to lose weight slowly.
- Set realistic goals.
- Like your body.
- Feel good about yourself.
- Recognize and accept your female factors.
- Have your body composition analyzed.
- Know your fat statistics.
- Get started!

Chapter Five

■

GETTING STARTED: DESIGNING YOUR 3-MONTH **OFF** PLAN

IF YOU are like most of my clients, this thought process (or something similar) is going on in your mind right now: "All of this makes sense to me. I believe in the OFF Plan. I'm ready to take it slowly and realistically. I'm ready to start, but how do I get started?"

The 3-month OFF Plan is just the tool you need to get started. It will provide the skills, guidance, structure, accountability, and evaluation to permanently outsmart your female fat cells. Why a 3-month program? Because in my experience, it takes most women about three months to begin the change process, to have a positive impact on their habits, and to see a measurable change in their bodies. After three months, you will realize that the OFF Plan *does* work and will gain the motivation to continue with the program for the next three months, the next year, the rest of your life.

Each of you will experience some measurable change in three months, but the length of time it will take to reach your ultimate goal will depend on you. Keep in mind that every woman is different; some women may respond quickly, while others may find their fat cells particularly stubborn. For example, Denise experienced substantial changes within two months, but Jennifer did not see major changes until the eighth month. Denise had never dieted and had never been pregnant. Jennifer had a child, was on the pill, was a nocturnal eater, and had been on eight diets in the past three years.

The greater the number of factors you have that activate your fat cells, the longer it will take to outsmart them. Remember, fat cells are smart and have memory. They remember the midnight snacks you've been eating, that fad diet you tried last January, and the diet pills you took three years ago. *It took you a while to develop habits that switched your fat cells on, give yourself time to switch them off. It takes patience and perseverance to fool a female fat cell.*

The 3-month OFF Plan is for *all* women of *all* ages at *all* stages of their lives. Of course, it's the ideal program for professional dieters and overeaters, but it is equally important for women who want to prevent future weight gain or may be struggling with their weight for the first time in their lives: Women who have gained five pounds on the pill; those whose metabolism has slowed down during menopause; those who have had an injury that affected their mobility; and women whose goal is to achieve their prepregnancy weight.

Lori, who is five feet tall, thought it would be impossible to get back to her, prepregnancy weight of ninety-two pounds. She had never had a weight problem until she gained forty-five pounds (almost 50 percent of her body weight) during her first pregnancy. While making an appointment, she told me that she would find it extremely difficult to diet. She loved food and refused to give up anything. She was pleasantly shocked when I responded "perfect." By following the OFF Plan for three months, she was encouraged by the way her body responded, and she was one pound below her prepregnancy weight within ten months. She was so happy that she sent me flowers and said she would give me a call after she had her second child.

The OFF Plan is for all women regardless of age and physiology, but you must tailor it to your needs and make it work for *you.* Before you can effectively switch your fat cells off, you must become aware of the factors in your lifestyle that have switched them on. The following questionnaires for each of the 6 OFF strategies will help you gain a greater awareness of yourself, your exercise habits, and your eating habits. You will then be able to use this increased awareness to prioritize the OFF strategies and focus on those most important for you.

STRATEGY #1: Do You Need to Aerobicize Your Fat Cells?

Rate the following statements as follows:

0—Never, 1—Seldom, 2—Frequently, 3—Always

1. I would rather diet than exercise.	____
2. I dislike exercise.	____
3. I gain weight when I exercise.	____
4. I don't have time to exercise.	____
5. I'll find any excuse not to exercise.	____
6. I try to exercise, but I'm not consistent.	____
7. I feel too fat to exercise.	____
8. I exercise to the point of exhaustion.	____
9. When I exercise, it's for less than 45 minutes.	____
10. I exercise so that I can eat more.	____
	TOTAL ____

Strategy #1: Aerobicize Your Fat Cells is the most important strategy!! Even if you scored 0 points, this strategy may help you tailor your exercise program to become more efficient in burning fat and turning off your female fat cells. If you scored 15 points or more, this strategy will help you to overcome your barriers to exercise, to be consistent with exercise, and to develop the best program for you and your body.

The common misconception is that "if you make a commitment to exercise for six weeks, you'll be motivated to continue because of the positive changes in your body." This may be true for men, but not for women. A three-month commitment is necessary to see measurable changes.

Don't worry—I will not ask you to start training for a marathon on day one of the program. As a matter of fact, you'll never have to exercise more than three times a week. Exercise is the first strategy because it is an ongoing strategy throughout the entire program. Over the next three months, we'll take it slowly and progressively build exercise into your life. Although it is the most important strategy because it is the only one that effectively releases fat from the fat cell (all the other strategies prevent fat storage), I also realize that it is the most difficult for women to schedule into their lives. But, difficult as it may be, it can be done!

Exercise is an old idea to which I will give new meaning. Like all the other strategies, we will relate exercise to changing the physiology of the female fat cell. As you will discover throughout the three-month program, there are special guidelines for women to use exercise effectively in outsmarting their fat cells. If you don't follow these special guidelines, you could be exercising every day for a year and still be waiting to see a change in your body. Jody came to see me after six months of exercise and no weight loss. By making one change, increasing the duration from 25 minutes to 45 minutes, she experienced substantial change within one month.

STRATEGY #2: Do You Need to Stop Dieting and Start Eating?

Rate each of the following statements as follows:

0—Never, 1—Seldom, 2—Frequently, 3—Always

1. I count calories. ____
2. I'm either on a diet or off a diet. ____
3. I eat diet foods. ____
4. I feel out of control with food. ____
5. Dieting is more important than good nutrition. ____
6. I start my diets on Mondays. ____
7. I eat for emotional reasons. ____
8. Hunger is a foreign feeling to me. ____
9. I wait until I am extremely hungry before I eat. ____
10. I eat to prevent hunger. ____
    TOTAL ____

If you scored 15 or more points, *Strategy #2: Stop Dieting and Start Eating*, will help you to give up dieting once and for all. More importantly, it will teach you how to eat again. Many women are afraid to give themselves permission to eat because they fear weight gain. Have no fear— you have to eat to lose weight, but you have to learn to eat when you are hungry. In my experience, most people eat in response to hunger only 10 percent to 20 percent of the time.

Over the years, food has acquired medicinal properties and special powers to nurture our emotions. We eat when we are depressed, stressed, bored, tired, lonely, anxious, etc. Over the years, we have also been conditioned to eat for social and environmental reasons that have nothing to do with hunger. Strategy #2 will help you to trust yourself to eat, to teach you to eat because of biological hunger (instead of social or emotional hunger), and to redefine what food means to you.

STRATEGY #3: Do You Need to Feed Your Body, Not Your Fat Cells?

Rate each of the following statements as follows:

0—Never, 1—Seldom, 2—Frequently, 3—Always

1. I feel uncomfortably full after I eat.   ____
2. I clean my plate.   ____
3. I eat quickly.   ____
4. I divide food into two categories, "good" and "bad." ____
5. When I eat "bad" foods, I feel guilty.   ____
6. I restrict "bad" foods and deprive myself.   ____
7. If a food says "diet," I eat as much as I want. ____
8. I overeat healthful foods.   ____
9. I overeat at restaurants and special events.   ____
10. I eat standing up.   ____

                                      TOTAL ____

If you scored 15 or more points, put special emphasis into *Strategy #3 Feed Your Body, Not Your Fat Cells*. It will help you to eat a wide variety of foods—moderately. Overeating means eating more calories than your body needs at a given time to function. Whenever you are overeating, you are feeding your fat cells. Those excess calories, whether they are from iceberg lettuce or ice cream, are not needed by your body, so they are stored in your fat cells. You may overeat for many reasons: sometimes simply from habit, and other times because you are socially conditioned. Do you give yourself permission to overeat when . . . ?

- You're at a party.
- You're at a party and do not want to offend the host.
- You're at a restaurant.
- You're at a restaurant and want to get your money's worth.
- You're watching TV.
- You're watching TV, and a food commercial comes on.
- You're in the kitchen.
- You're in the kitchen preparing dinner.
- You're celebrating your birthday.
- You're celebrating someone else's birthday.

Feeding your body does not mean eating low-calorie diet foods such as salads and carrot sticks. It means eating a wide variety of foods in moderation when you are hungry. There are no "good" or "bad" foods in the OFF Plan. All food choices are created equal as long as you are feeding your body.

This strategy is extremely important. You could be following all the other strategies, but if you're overeating, you are feeding your fat cells, and you may never see a change in your body.

STRATEGY #4: Do You Need to Shrink and Multiply Your Meals?

Rate each of the statements as follows:

0—Never, 1—Seldom, 2—Frequently, 3—Always

1. I skip breakfast. _____
2. I skip lunch. _____
3. I eat three balanced meals a day. _____
4. I avoid snacking. _____
5. When I snack, I choose "junk" foods. _____
6. If I'm going out to dinner, I eat little that day. _____
7. I would rather eat food than throw it away. _____
8. I feel uncomfortably full after lunch. _____
9. I feel uncomfortably full after dinner. _____
10. A meal includes meat, vegetable, starch, salad, and dessert. _____

TOTAL _____

If you scored 15 or more points, *Strategy #4: Shrink and Multiply Your Meals*, will help you to prevent overeating at meals and to supply your body with a constant source of calories throughout the day—without storing any in your fat cells. I know that society has led us to believe that snacking is "bad" and three balanced meals a day is "good." But could society be wrong about eating right?

Snacking can and should be a healthy part of your diet. When I asked Jenny to define snacking, she said, "It's eating a candy bar at 3:30 P.M. for a pick-me-up and a pint of ice cream at night while watching TV." We have equated snacking with junk food. Snacking is only detrimental if you eat when you are not hungry, and if you overeat. When I then asked Jenny to define a balanced meal, she said, "Well, it contains all the food groups plus dessert. It includes meat, vegetable, starch, salad, bread, milk, and dessert." Eating this traditional balanced meal is overeating.

This strategy will help you to change your view of snacks

versus meals and give you the skills to eat smaller, more frequent meals throughout the day.

STRATEGY #5: Do You Need to Become a Daytime Eater?

Rate each of the following statements as follows:

0—Never, 1—Seldom, 2—Frequently, 3—Always

1. I eat late at night.   _____
2. I eat before going to bed.   _____
3. I snack while watching TV at night.   _____
4. Dinner is my biggest meal of the day.   _____
5. I eat dinner after 6:00 p.m.   _____
6. I binge at night when I am alone.   _____
7. I raid the refrigerator in the middle of the night. _____
8. I restrain my eating during the day, then overeat
   at night.   _____
9. The first thing I do when I get home from work or my
   day's activities is eat.   _____
10. Eating helps me to relax at night.   _____
                                                                  TOTAL _____

If you scored 15 points or more, *Strategy #5: Become a Daytime Eater*, will help you to transfer some of your "night" calories to "day" calories. Your metabolism is slowest at night, so the more you eat at night, the more will be stored in your fat cells.

If you are a typical American, about 70 percent of your food is eaten after 5:00 P.M. Other societies eat their largest meal during the day—and they do not have as much of a weight problem. We are nocturnal eaters, and we *do* have a weight problem. We not only eat our largest meal at dinner but also top it off with nighttime grazing. When Sara asked, "Should I eat my hot meal for lunch and have a bowl of soup for dinner?" she had gotten the message.

STRATEGY #6: Do You Need to Fat-Proof Your Diet?

Rate each of the statements as follows:

0—Never, 1—Seldom, 2—Frequently, 3—Always

1. I love the taste of fat. _____
2. I add butter or margarine to my food. _____
3. I use oils in cooking. _____
4. I put mayonnaise on my sandwiches. _____
5. I eat out in fast-food restaurants. _____
6. I eat deep-fried foods. _____
7. When I read food labels, I look for the calorie content, not the fat content. _____
8. I feel margarine is a better choice than butter. _____
9. I'm more concerned about cholesterol than fat in my diet. _____
10. If a food says "reduced fat," I buy it. _____

TOTAL _____

If you scored 15 points or more, your diet is most likely high in fat. *Strategy #6: Fat-Proof Your Diet* will help you to choose lower fat foods and recondition your taste buds.

Although it is your eating habits that have the most influence on the female fat cell, fat in your diet is more likely to become fat in your fat cell. The higher the fat content of your diet, the bigger your fat cells.

This strategy is the last one for a reason. In most "diet" plans, food choices are the primary focus. Not in the OFF Plan. The eating-habit strategies come first, the food-choice strategy comes second. And the *only* recommendation for food choices is to reduce your fat intake. There is no mention of eliminating or even reducing starches and sugars. Starches (breads, potatoes, pasta, etc.) are fattening only when you overeat them or load them with butter. Sugars are only fattening when you overeat them. Fat can be fattening whether you overeat it or not.

TAILORING THE OFF PLAN
TO YOUR NEEDS

To tailor the **OFF** Plan to your specific needs, you must determine which strategies will be most important for *you*. Note your scores from the previous questionnaires, then list the strategies from highest to lowest scores.

WHAT WERE YOUR SCORES?   **SCORE**

Strategy #1: Aerobicize Your Fat Cells   _____

Strategy #2: Stop Dieting and Start Eating   _____

Strategy #3: Feed Your Body, Not Your Fat Cells   _____

Strategy #4: Shrink and Multiply Your Meals   _____

Strategy #5: Become a Daytime Eater   _____

Strategy #6: Fat-Proof Your Diet   _____

LIST THE STRATEGIES FROM HIGHEST SCORE
TO LOWEST SCORE:

1. _____
2. _____
3. _____
4. _____
5. _____
6. _____

Did you find:
- That all strategies are of equal importance?
- That some strategies will be more important than others?
- That you are already following some of the strategies?
- That you have become more aware of your habits?

By ranking the strategies from highest to lowest score, you have identified the strategies that will be most effective for you. All 6 of the strategies are important to outsmart your fat cells and do work together in switching your fat cells off, but it is important to tailor the program to your specific needs. The strategies with the highest scores will be the strategies that require the most attention and effort in order to integrate them into your lifestyle.

Scoring low on a strategy doesn't mean that you can neglect it and move on to the next one. All the strategies build upon one another, and each is necessary for success. Scoring low means that you are already practicing some positive behaviors, and you'll use that strategy to reinforce and fine-tune those positive behaviors.

Whatever your scores, it is unrealistic to think that you must follow all 6 of the OFF strategies 100 percent of the time. Unlike dieting, the OFF Action Plan is not "all or nothing"—it is flexible and sensible. With today's busy lifestyle and schedules, circumstances can change on a day-to-day basis. The OFF Plan can change with you. It takes the long-term view where the *average* is the key to success, not short-term bursts of willpower.

Now that you have a greater awareness of your exercise habits, your eating habits, and your needs, let me give you a preview of what's to come.

The next three months will be broken down into two-week segments. Each two-week period has a strategy #1 exercise focus, another eating habit strategy focus, and also continues to build upon the strategies from the previous weeks. By the end of three months, you will have slowly and progressively implemented all of the 6 strategies.

THE 3-MONTH OFF ACTION PLAN

WEEKS	STRATEGY FOCUS					
	#1	#2	#3	#4	#5	#6
1 & 2	X	X				
3 & 4	X	X	X			
5 & 6	X	X	X	X		
7 & 8	X	X	X	X	X	
9 & 10	X	X	X	X	X	X
11 & 12	X	X	X	X	X	X

These strategies have not been randomly numbered and placed in the pyramid structure. Exercise is the first strategy and an ongoing one for the entire three months because it is the most important in outsmarting your female fat cells. The remaining five strategies target positive eating habits, and their sequence makes sense and actually should occur naturally. When you stop dieting, you need to start eating. When you start eating, you need to learn to eat moderately by feeding your body, not your fat cells. When you start eating moderately, you'll find that you are eating smaller, more frequent meals. Then you take those smaller meals and eat more of them during the day. Then you choose lower-fat foods for those smaller, daytime meals. See, it makes sense.

Now, let's discuss the exercise strategy a bit more. It is a little different from the other strategies because it is a focus of each of the two-week segments. The reason for this is that aerobic exercise is vital to the success of the program, and it's the strategy that requires the most commitment and is also the most difficult.

To ease your way into exercise without deemphasizing its importance, each two-week segment slowly builds exercise into your life and enhances your fat-burning potential. If you've got the "I'd rather diet than exercise" attitude or have a busy schedule that has prevented you from exercising, this approach should relax you a bit. Think of how many times you've said to yourself, "I should start exercising," but you haven't, or if you have, you're lucky if you have made it through a week or two. Making the commitment and finding the time to exercise can be so overwhelming that it paralyzes you.

That's why *this* time you are going to ease into exercise. You'll start exercising just once a week, then twice a week, and so on—but you'll never have to do it more than three times a week. Throughout the program, each two-week segment will slowly increase the number of times a week and the number of minutes spent exercising. In the first month, you'll condition your fat cells to release fat by activating the lipolytic enzymes. Then, in the next two months, you'll achieve your full fat-burning potential. After the three months, I hope you'll be hooked (or at least more accepting), and then we'll put on the final touches to "aerobicize your fat cells with a new attitude" in Chapter 12.

If aerobic exercise is already a part of your life, congratulations! You'll skip the motivation and commitment-building and get right into your maximum fat-burning potential.

As I have mentioned, each two-week period has an exercise focus plus an eating habit strategy focus with specific goals within that strategy to achieve. The following chapters will go into greater detail on goal-setting and techniques to achieve those goals. But, to let you know where we are headed, here is a brief description of the next three months.

WEEKS 1 & 2

OFF Strategy Focus: Stop Dieting and Start Eating

OFF Goals:
1. Give up dieting and the diet mentality.
2. Identify your hunger signals and learn to eat when you are hungry.
3. Select an exercise you enjoy (tolerate?) and do it once a week for 10 to 15 minutes at a moderate intensity.
4. If you are already exercising, don't cut down to once a week—continue what you are doing, but make sure that you are in your fat-burning zone.

WEEKS 3 & 4

OFF Strategy Focus: Feed Your Body, Not Your Fat Cells

OFF Goals:
1. Continue with the goals from weeks 1 & 2.
2. Learn to eat whatever you want without guilt as long as you don't overeat.

3. Identify your fullness signals and learn to stop eating when comfortable, not full.

4. Add another day of exercise a week (or two if you are ready) and slowly increase the duration to 20 minutes each session.

WEEKS 5 & 6

OFF Strategy Focus: Shrink and Multiply Your Meals

OFF Goals:
1. Continue with the goals from weeks 1–4.
2. Learn to eat and enjoy smaller, more frequent meals throughout the day.
3. Plan your day with mini-meals and maxi-snacks.
4. Add one more day of exercise a week and increase the duration to 30 minutes each session.

WEEKS 7 & 8

OFF Strategy Focus: Become a Daytime Eater

OFF Goals:
1. Continue with the goals from weeks 1–6.
2. Match your eating to your metabolism by consuming more of your calories during the day and less at night.
3. Learn to control your nighttime snacking.
4. Exercise three times a week (if you get the urge for a fourth day, go for it), and increase the duration to 35 minutes each session.

WEEKS 9 & 10

OFF Strategy Focus: Fat-Proof Your Diet

OFF Goals:
1. Continue with the goals from weeks 1–8.
2. Reduce your fat intake to 20 percent of calories by balancing your food choices.
3. Identify the fat content of foods by reading food labels and finding the hidden fat.
4. Exercise three times a week (four or five if you want) and increase the duration to 40 minutes each session.

WEEKS 11 & 12

OFF Strategy Focus: All Strategies: Taking the **OFF** Plan on the Road

OFF Goals:
1. Continue with the goals from weeks 1–10.
2. Practice all of the strategies together.
3. Practice the strategies during special occasions: holidays, dining out, vacations.
4. Exercise three times a week (four or five if you want) and increase the duration to 45 minutes each session.
5. Evaluate changes in your eating and exercise habits.
6. Evaluate changes in your fat statistics.

This is what your program generally will look like for the next three months. Some of you may move more quickly than I have suggested, others may find that they are working on all the strategies together, and still others may find that they do not need such a structured program (but rare is the person who requires no structure). What is most important is that the program suits your needs. You all have different eating and exercising habits, you all scored differently on the assessment questionnaires, and you all have different lifestyles. Tailor the program to your specific needs. The first three months of the OFF Plan are to give you guidance on how to make changes in your behaviors. Eventually, it stops being a "plan" and becomes the way you are.

I encourage you to read each of the following chapters, stop, and practice the target strategy for two weeks. I realize that you will be tempted to read through the entire book. If that is the case, go back to Chapter 6, Weeks 1 & 2, and really start the program.

I have provided a plan of action for a proven successful program, but it's up to you to put that plan into action, to achieve the defined goals, and to tailor it to your needs. You've prepared yourself. You've identified those strategies most important for you. You know how to get started with the 3-month OFF Plan. Now, it's up to you to outsmart your female fat cells with the following chapters—they are your stepping stones to success. Good Luck!!

Chapter Six

■

WEEKS 1 & 2:
STOP DIETING
AND START EATING

"WHAT?! YOU actually want me to eat? What kind of diet is this?" That's the point—it's not a diet. I want you to give up dieting once and for all and learn how to eat again. Women have been struggling not to eat for most of their lives. I want you to give up the endless struggle and give yourself the *freedom to eat when you are hungry*.

Trusting yourself to eat may be a terrifying step into the unknown. However, as scary as it might seem, you have to eat regularly to lose weight. As discussed in Chapter 2, "You Can't Starve a Fat Cell," dieting only serves to activate your fat survival mechanism, make your fat cells larger, and make them more efficient in storage. Remember our anti-dieting motto: "If you want to gain weight, go on a diet." To briefly review, if you restrict calories, your metabolism slows down to survive on a fewer number of calories. The less you eat, the fewer calories your body needs, the more calories your fat cells store, and the more you weigh. It's a downward cycle of eating less and weighing more.

The average woman today eats about 200 fewer calories and weighs about six pounds more than the average woman in 1960. She's also been on at least ten diets over the last thirty years or so. I know it doesn't make sense that you can eat less and weigh more. But dieting itself doesn't make sense because the end result is weight gain, not weight loss.

If a few months go by, and you don't go on a diet, your fat cells start wondering if you are still alive. They were anxiously awaiting your next diet, all geared up and ready to do battle for fat protection—but, you did something different. You didn't go on a diet. They were ready for starvation, but you didn't starve, you kept eating. Eventually, they will realize that starvation is not pending and will inactivate the fat-survival mechanism and will turn off the fat-storing lipogenic enzymes.

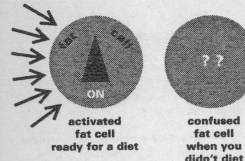

activated	confused	inactivated
fat cell	fat cell	fat cell when
ready for a diet	when you	you give up
	didn't diet	dieting forever

If you want to gain weight, I encourage you to go on and off diets for the rest of your life. *If you want to lose weight, you have to eat and exercise.* But before I discuss the importance of eating to weight loss, I want to reemphasize the effects of dieting on weight gain with Susan's case. Her daughter was getting married in six weeks, and she waited until the last minute to lose her excess twenty-five pounds. She made an appointment with me expecting to be put on a strict diet. I shared with her my philosophy of slowly outsmarting her fat cells and explained why a quick weight loss would simply fuel her fat cells. Susan didn't care what happened to her fat cells as long as she lost the weight in time for the wedding, so she left my office in search of a "guaranteed quick weight loss." Before I let her out of my office, I took some measurements and asked her to come back after she lost the twenty-five pounds. She also came back to see me after she had gone back to her old eating habits and gained back the twenty-five pounds plus some. Here is what happened to Susan:

	Pre-diet	Diet	Post-diet
Weight (pounds)	175	150	179
Percentage of body fat	34%	30%	41%
Pounds of fat	60	45	74
Pounds of muscle	115	105	105

Susan's fat cells were switched on. She was only four pounds heavier than her prediet weight, but she had fourteen pounds more fat on her body and ten pounds less muscle. Her body sacrificed muscle while on the diet and gained fat when she went off the diet. The increased fat mass and reduced muscle mass meant that fewer calories were burned and more calories were stored. Fat stores, and muscle burns. Remember, muscle is metabolically active tissue that requires calories to function. The less muscle you have, the fewer calories you burn. You do not want to lose muscle unless your goal is a slower metabolism.

In case you were wondering what ultimately happened with Susan, she did switch her fat cells off with the OFF Plan. She lost the fourteen pounds of fat gained as a result of the diet plus an additional fifteen pounds of fat. Nevertheless, the previous dieting situation had made her fat cells smarter and stronger.

I hope that by now you have decided to stop dieting once and for all. You certainly have extensive knowledge of the unhealthy truth about dieting, but sometimes knowledge isn't enough. Debra started dieting at age five when her mother first dragged her to a diet doctor. "I've been to fat farms, weight-loss camps, and to every diet program across the country. Dieting is a part of my life, a part of me. If I stop dieting, I won't know who I am." If you are like Debra, the more diets you have been on, the more difficult they may be to give up. Dieting is as much a part of some women's lives as brushing their teeth. It's something that they automatically do the first Monday of every month.

If you can't decide to stop dieting today, perhaps you first need to give up the diet mentality. The diet mentality is a state of mind that controls your thoughts and behaviors. It's the combination of all the beliefs and attitudes that have formed in our dieting society—the calorie obsessions, the diet foods, the deprivation, the restrictions. It's the belief that "you can't control your eating and lose weight unless you diet." The reality is you can't control your eating and lose weight unless you do *not* diet.

There are many beliefs that clients have shared with me that have no basis in reality and border on the ridiculous, but they keep us caught up in the fantasy of dieting:

- If you eat a candy bar with a diet soft drink, they cancel each other out.
- If no one sees you eat it, it has no calories.
- The leftovers on your kid's plate are devoid of calories.
- If you eat it out of the bag or the box, the calories don't count.
- If you eat standing up, you burn away the calories.
- As long as you eat "diet" foods, you won't gain weight.

Obviously, much of the diet mentality, irrational thoughts, and fantasy beliefs has to do with calories and the hope that calories will miraculously disappear. You may have memorized the calorie content of 100,000 foods, but all you've done is occupied valuable brain space. You may even have burned a few extra calories in the memorization process, but you haven't burned any fat. A calorie is a calorie only in a test tube. You are not a test tube. You are a unique individual with a special genetic structure, biochemistry, and metabolism. Your body utilizes calories differently from mine, your friend's, your sister's, your boss's.

You may have been told that you need X number of calories a day. If you eat too many, you'll gain weight. If you eat too few, you'll lose weight. This may be true on paper or in a test tube, but not in your body. Calories do not count. What counts is *how* you eat those calories and *where* they come from: carbohydrates, protein, or fat.

Because of our obsession with calorie-counting, we have also become diet-food-dependent. Many of my clients won't eat a food unless it has "diet" plastered all over it. Then, because it says "diet," they think that they can eat as much of it as they want to without gaining weight. Wrong! Only your mind knows it is a diet food, your body doesn't.

So, there's the "stop dieting" part of this strategy: Realize that counting calories and eating diet foods only feed (so to speak) into the diet mentality. If you need to further convince yourself that diets do not work, reread Chapter 2, "You Can't Starve a Fat Cell."

Now for the "start eating" part . . .

When I told Stephanie, "If you are really serious about losing weight, you have to start eating more," she thought I was losing my mind. She had been steadily cutting calories over the years so that she was eating about 800 calories a day—and gaining weight because her fat cells had become extremely efficient at storing and her metabolism had slowed down. No one believed her. Her doctor thought she was a closet eater, and her husband accused her of eating boxes of Twinkies at work. The reality was that she was gaining weight on salad and carrots.

My goal was to get Stephanie to eat. I slowly increased her food intake to give her metabolism a boost and fool her fat cells. Eating an extra piece of bread or an apple wasn't enough for her to gain weight, but it was enough to bring her body out of the starvation/fat protection mode. Within a year she was losing weight and eating about 1,500 calories a day. Stephanie's is an extreme case, but it emphasizes how vital eating is to your metabolism and weight loss. *You have to eat to lose weight.*

I want to help you gain the trust in yourself to *eat without guilt when you are hungry*. The problem is most people eat when they are not hungry. When I was in college, I did an eye-opening survey on why people eat. I stood on a street corner and asked people of different shapes and sizes, "Why do you eat?" The fit and lean people looked at me with bewilderment and quickly answered "because I'm hungry." The unfit and overweight people delivered a ten-minute monologue on a multitude of emotional and social reasons for eating. Over 50 percent of them didn't even mention hunger.

Ask yourself, "Why do I eat?" to become aware of all the reasons (excuses?) for putting food into your mouth. Here are some of my clients' favorite reasons:

1. *I-Deserve-It Eating.* You spent two hours in bumper-to-bumper traffic; that has to be worth at least two candy bars. You just completed a big project, you deserve your favorite meal at your favorite restaurant.
2. *The Last Supper Syndrome.* This may be the last time you'll ever see cheesecake for the rest of your life; you better eat it now while you have the chance.
3. *Nobody's Around.* They are finally gone, now you can eat the cake without the dirty looks and remarks. You can now enter the world of uninhibited closet eating.
4. *Kitchen Eating.* You walked in the kitchen, but you don't remember why. While you are there, you might as well open the cupboard and see what there is to eat.
5. *See Food Eating.* It's sitting there on the counter; you see it, you eat it. It's as simple as that.
6. *What-the-Hell Eating.* You ate too much at lunch and now there is an office birthday party. What-the-hell, you blew it at lunch anyway, might as well have a piece or two of birthday cake.
7. *Preventive Eating.* You're not hungry now, but you may be in an hour and what if there is no food around? You'd better eat now just in case.

8. *Quick-Fix Eating.* You're feeling depressed, lonely, sad. You need a quick fix to make yourself feel better. Ice cream has had medicinal properties since childhood.

Most people eat in response to hunger only about 20 percent of the time. They eat when they are not hungry 80 percent of the time. If you eat when you are not hungry, your body doesn't need it, and it goes straight to your fat cells. If you eat when you are hungry, your body needs the calories and they bypass the fat cells. As you begin the eating process, you *can* and *should* eat when you are hungry.

To begin the process of knowing when you are hungry and then eating without guilt, the Hunger/Fullness Rating Scale is a valuable tool. I recommend recording your hunger every hour or so to become aware of all your stages of hunger and fullness. It is important to note that what you're eating is of no concern in regard to eating when you are hungry.

The **OFF** Hunger/Fullness Rating Scale

10 - Absolutely, positively, lie-on-the-floor stuffed
 9 - So full that you are starting to hurt
 8 - Very full and bloated
 7 - Starting to feel uncomfortable
 6 - Slightly overeating
 5 - Perfectly comfortable
 4 - First signal that your body needs food
 3 - Strong signals to eat
 2 - Very hungry, irritable
 1 - Extreme hunger, dizziness

If you are above level 4, you are not hungry, and your body doesn't need food. You may feel a "need" of some kind and interpret it as a need for food, but the only thing you accomplish is bigger fat cells. Maybe what you really need is a hug, a nap, or a cry. Give yourself what you really need.

As long as you experience hunger, your body needs food.

You do want to experience hunger, but not extreme hunger. The OFF Plan chart differs from other hunger-rating charts that recommend waiting until you are at level 1 (or 0) before you can eat. I believe this can be disastrous. When you are this hungry, you are overhungry—so hungry that it causes you to lose control of your eating. You'll overeat, feel guilty, then think about dieting again. Being too hungry is the start of starvation.

At level 3 or 4, your body is sending you signals that it needs food and you need to eat. It is letting you know that you can and should eat without guilt. *What are your body's signals of hunger?*

As you begin using this hunger-rating scale, you will come to know the difference between head hunger and body hunger. Head hunger is when your emotions and your environment control why and when you eat, not your body. Head hunger is when you look at the clock, it says noontime, and you think, "It's time to eat," but your body may not think so. To help distinguish between the two, continually ask yourself, *"Am I really hungry?"* and assess how your body feels. As you get used to this question, you'll find that often you are not feeling hunger, you are feeling emotions—anxiety, depression, anger. Get in touch with the biological hunger signals that are submerged beneath your emotional signals.

As you are getting acquainted with your biological hunger signals, it is easy to confuse hunger signals with thirst signals. If you drink water only when you are thirsty, you'll consume only about 50 percent of the fluids your body needs. For some reason, our thirst mechanisms are faulty. If you think you are hungry, it may be your body trying to inform you that it needs fluids, not food. To be sure, put your hunger to the water test: Drink a glass of water, wait fifteen minutes, then check in with your body to see if you were really hungry. After satisfying your thirst needs, you may find that it wasn't hunger after all.

Also, by drinking water throughout the day and adequately hydrating your body, you'll be more confident that the signals are true hunger signals. How many glasses of water should you drink a day? "Oh, oh, I know!! Eight a day!" Usually everyone thinks they know the answer to this question. It is in every nutrition book, every diet program, every health club, but the funny thing is that no one really knows. As a matter of fact, if you did some research on the subject or asked your doctor where the eight-glass recommendation came from, you wouldn't find an answer. Many people try drinking eight glasses a day, spend half the time in the bathroom, and feel like they are drowning. If eight glasses seems like too much, maybe six glasses is the right answer for you, or five. My doctor's recommendation is to drink enough water so that your urine is clear in color. It's only a suggestion, but check out the color of your urine.

Not only may thirst trigger false hunger, but sugar may also do the same. Don't worry, I will never even come close to suggesting that you eliminate sugar from your diet. But I am going to recommend that when you eat sugar foods make sure that it is not on an empty stomach. Let me explain.

It's 3:30 in the afternoon, you know that you are experiencing real hunger, and you go for a handful of jelly beans. Jelly beans are 100 percent sugar, and are quickly digested and absorbed into your bloodstream. Within ten to fifteen minutes your blood sugar will rise dramatically. That may give you an initial burst of energy with the sugar high, but the sugar high is always followed by the sugar low. Insulin is secreted when blood sugar levels are high, and it transfers sugar from your blood into your cells. Blood sugar levels drop within the next ten to fifteen minutes, which can make you feel hungry. But how can you really be hungry when you ate the jelly beans just thirty minutes ago? That is not true hunger.

If you had eaten the jelly beans with your sandwich at lunch, you would not experience the drop in blood sugar. There is starch in the bread and protein in the meat that will slow the digestion and absorption of sugar, minimize the sugar high, and prevent the sugar low. *When you eat sugar, make sure it is with a meal.*

If you use artificial sweeteners, I also suggest consuming them with meals because they may stimulate a false sense of hunger in some people. If you drink artificially sweetened iced tea, your taste buds are stimulated and send a message to the brain that sugar is on its way, even though it is not real sugar. Your brain is excited in anticipation of the sugar and thinks that blood sugar will be rising any minute, so it sends the message to secrete insulin. Insulin takes sugar from your blood and transports it into your cells. By the time your brain realizes "This isn't sugar, it's fake stuff," some insulin may have already been secreted. The end result is a drop in blood sugar, which may stimulate appetite.

Knowing when you are hungry and eating when you are hungry is the first step in outsmarting your female fat cells. Trust your body and give yourself permission to eat when you are hungry.

Now that you have all the background to Stop Dieting and Start Eating, let's put this strategy into practice . . .

YOUR OFF ACTION PLAN: WEEKS 1 & 2

OFF Strategy Focus: Stop Dieting and Start Eating

      OFF Goals: 1. Give up dieting and the dieting mentality.
                2. Identify your hunger signals and learn to eat when you are hungry.
                3. Select an exercise you enjoy (tolerate?) and do it once a week for 10 to 15 minutes at a moderate intensity.
                4. If you are already exercising, don't cut down to once a week—continue what you are doing, but make sure that you are in your fat-burning zone.

OFF Techniques:
                1. Analyze your diet mentality.

2. Identify your beliefs about counting calories and diet foods.
3. Reread Chapter 2, "You Can't Starve a Fat Cell."
4. Identify your emotional eating triggers.
5. Identify your social eating triggers.
6. Use the hunger-rating scale.
7. Identify your true biological hunger signals.
8. Ask yourself, "Am I hungry? What do I need?"
9. Put your hunger to the water test.
10. Adequately hydrate your body.
11. Avoid sugar on an empty stomach.
12. Avoid artificial sweeteners on an empty stomach.
13. **Keep hunger records for two weeks to practice these techniques.**

You may have been asked to keep food records before, but this one is different: It's a hunger record, not a food record. You will not be asked to count calories; you will be asked to rate your hunger.

I recommend that you record your hunger every hour or so to discover your true biological hunger signals and to get in tune with those signals. Then record if you ate and why you ate. Here is an example:

HUNGER/FULLNESS RECORDS
TO START EATING

TIME	HUNGER LEVEL	DID YOU EAT?	WHY DID YOU OR DIDN'T YOU EAT?
6:00 am	5	no	not hungry, too early
7:00 am	4	yes	a little hungry
8:00 am	5	no	not hungry
9:00 am	5	no	not hungry
10:00 am	4	no	too busy to eat
11:00 am	3	no	it's almost lunchtime
12:00 pm	2	yes	Starving!
1:00 pm	7	no	too full from lunch
2:00 pm	6	no	not hungry
3:00 pm	5	yes	felt I needed an energy boost
4:00 pm	5	no	not hungry
5:00 pm	4	no	no food around
6:00 pm	4	no	riding the bus
7:00 pm	3	yes	hungry - dinner's ready
8:00 pm	6	no	watching TV
9:00 pm	5	yes	bored with TV show
10:00 pm	7	no	full, tired, bedtime

These food records focus only on hunger and the reasons for eating. I don't care what you ate or how much you ate, for right now—just if you ate and why you ate. There is a blank food record on the following page for you to use as a guideline, but some clients find that designing their own record in a small notebook is most realistic. They keep it handy in their purse or briefcase and can bring it anywhere.

If you are already eating when you are hungry, then reinforce your positive behaviors and focus on not letting yourself get too hungry. Everyone can benefit from becoming more conscious of their hunger signals. It is the first step in outsmarting your female fat cells.

YOUR FIRST STEP IN AEROBICIZING YOUR FAT CELLS

The major difference between this exercise program and others that you may have tried (and failed at) in the past is that today you are going to take only the *first step*. You will not start by exercising every day or even every other day—just one day each week over the next two weeks. Now that's truly a nonthreatening first step.

As I have mentioned earlier in this book, aerobic exercise is a focus of every two-week segment because it is more important than any other strategy in outsmarting your female fat cells. It's the only one that will stimulate the fat-releasing lipolytic enzymes. There is no food you can eat, no pill you can take, no cream that you can rub on that will activate the releasing enzymes. Only aerobic exercise will do it.

HUNGER/FULLNESS RECORDS
TO START EATING

TIME	HUNGER LEVEL	DID YOU EAT?	WHY DID YOU OR DIDN'T YOU EAT?

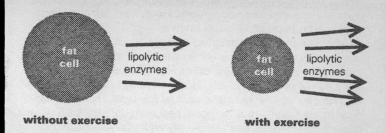

without exercise   **with exercise**

The first step will be to condition your fat cells to release fat. As a matter of fact, we'll call the entire first month the conditioning month. You probably won't be releasing much fat in the first two weeks or the first month, but you will be creating a fat-releasing environment. Your fat cells are stubborn and don't know how to release fat. You need the enzymes before you can release fat, and you need to teach your fat cells how to use the enzymes to release fat.

What kind of exercise will stimulate the lipolytic enzymes? Only aerobic exercise. Aerobic means "with oxygen," and a constant supply of oxygen is necessary to release fat.

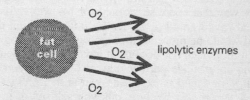

It never fails that a client bows her head in embarrassment and asks me, "Is walking okay?" Yes, walking is a great exercise because it is aerobic. Any exercise is aerobic if it uses your major muscle groups (buttocks and thighs) in a rhythmical, nonstop movement. Walking fits the criteria, so does jogging, rowing, climbing stairs, cross-country skiing, swimming, jumping rope, aerobic dance classes, aqua-aerobics classes, step classes, and rollerskating. One of my clients even tried rollerblading—and loves it.

An exercise is not aerobic (called anaerobic) if it has stop/start movements and is not continuous. Tennis, golf, downhill skiing, and softball are examples of anaerobic exercises. They do not produce a steady increase in heart rate and breathing rate—so they are not significant fat releasers. However, they do stimulate your muscle mass and metabolism, so if you enjoy these activities, don't stop—just add an aerobic activity.

So, which aerobic exercise are you going to choose? As long as it is aerobic, all types of exercise are created equal. In your decision-making process, please consider your lifestyle, work schedule, and preferences.

- Do you like to exercise indoors or outdoors?
- Do you like to exercise alone or with a partner?
- Do you like group exercise programs?
- What day(s) of the week would be best for you?
- What time of day would be best for you?

"I don't like exercising indoors or outdoors, alone or with people, any time of any day." Maureen disliked exercise so much that she had a tough time rising above her negativism. The only way that exercise worked for her was by buying a dog she always wanted (a golden Lab) and walking the dog. Maybe it would be more accurate to say that the dog walked her, but it motivated her because it gave her enjoyment.

Finding an exercise partner may also provide some motivation. If your friend is expecting you at the 5:30 P.M. aerobics class, you're less likely to talk yourself out of it. If your co-worker is meeting you at the gym before work, you're less likely to hit the sleep button.

You have to enjoy it or at least tolerate it to do it. Please don't invest in an expensive piece of exercise equipment unless you know that you'll like it. There are countless people with exercise bikes and rowing machines that are collecting cobwebs in the garage. If you are not sure what you like to do, walking is the best start because it is inexpensive and you can do it anywhere. All you need is a good pair of walking shoes.

Make the first step in exercise as easy as possible. Choose a day when you know that you'll have the time. Choose a time of day that is convenient and fits into your schedule. If you choose to exercise at 5:30 A.M. and you've never been up before 6:00 A.M. in your life, the odds are better that you will win the lottery than make it out of bed. Maybe lunchtime or evening is the easiest right now. The time of day doesn't matter, what matters is that you do it.

First, exercise needs to be aerobic; second, it needs to be moderate. "You mean I don't have to feel like I'm going to have a heart attack?" Absolutely not. Your fat-releasing enzymes will be stimulated only if the exercise is moderate. Here's why: Both underexercising and overexercising result in an insufficient supply of oxygen to your fat cells. If you are taking a leisurely walk while window-shopping, your body is not pushed enough and your heart rate and breathing are not increased enough. If you are trying to break the world record for the fifty-yard dash, you are pushing your body too hard and you are out of breath. Only moderate exercise gives you a steady, increased heart rate and a steady supply of oxygen to your fat cells.

Most of my clients find that they have been overexercising. "If I'm going to exercise, I might as well push myself as hard as I can." That's the "no pain, no gain" attitude. If you are exercising too hard, you will not see a change in your body because

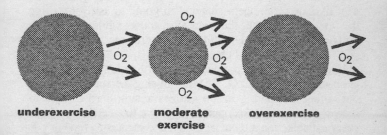

underexercise   moderate   overexercise
                        exercise

your lipolytic releasing enzymes haven't been activated. Instead of mobilizing fat for energy, your body uses sugar (and maybe a little muscle) because it is more readily available.

So how can you make sure that you are exercising moderately? There are a number of ways to assess whether or not you are releasing fat from your fat cells by exercising moderately. Typically, an equation or chart is used to determine your target heart rate.

If you choose, you can use this method, but it can be inaccurate and difficult to do. Most people have a tough time finding their pulse to begin with, and then they can't count, watch the clock, and walk at the same time. If you do choose to use the target - heart rate method to monitor your intensity, here is the equation:

$$(220 - \text{your age}) \times 60\% = \text{your low target}$$
$$(220 - \text{your age}) \times 75\% = \text{your high target}$$

For example, if you are 40 years old:

$$220 - 40 = 180 \times 60\% - 108 \text{ beats/minute}$$
$$220 - 40 = 180 \times 75\% - 135 \text{ beats/minute}$$

Target heart rate is between 108 and 135 beats/minute. To be in your moderate intensity, you want to make sure that your heart rate is within the range of your lower and upper target.

Instead of the above heart rate method, I'm going to share with you an easier and more accurate way that focuses on your rate of breathing. It's called the sing test. Whether you're tone deaf like me or an opera singer, I'm going to ask you to sing the first line of a song that everyone knows while you are exercising—"Old MacDonald." Bear with me a minute and you'll understand why I chose this song.

In case you don't remember, the first line is "Old MacDonald had a farm, E I E I O." If you can sing the entire line without taking a breath, you are not exercising hard enough to deliver the necessary oxygen. If you have to take a breath after every syllable, you are out of breath and exercising too hard. If you take three breaths evenly dispersed, then it's moderate.

Old MacDonald (breath) had a farm (breath), E I E I O (breath).

Because I love rating scales, I'm going to give you a third method to assess whether or not you are burning fat. This is a scale to determine how you feel and how hard you are exercising:

10 - Call an ambulance
 9 - Excruciatingly, painfully hard
 8 - Extremely hard, out of breath
 7 - Very hard, getting out of breath
 6 - Somewhat hard, you can sing
 5 - Moderately hard, you can sing
 4 - Slightly hard, you can sing
 3 - Easy, breathing not increased
 2 - Very easy, standing with little movement
 1 - Awake, but barely
 0 - State of blissful unconsciousness

At levels 4, 5, and 6 you are in your fat-burning range—it's not too easy or too hard, you can sing, and it's perfectly moderate. I recommend monitoring your exercise intensity with any of these methods about every five minutes. This will allow you to speed up or slow down as necessary during your workout.

"I get the moderate part, but how many minutes do you want me to do my moderate aerobic exercise?" For the first two weeks, I am most concerned that you do it, not necessarily how many minutes you do it. Let's strive for ten to fifteen minutes. If you want to do it longer—great! If you are already exercising, don't cut back to once a week for fifteen minutes, just make sure that you are exercising moderately to release fat. What's most important is that you go at your own pace; start slowly and work up to ten to fifteen minutes. Moderate exercise should never be painful. Your thighs should never feel like they went through a meat grinder. Your heart should never feel like it is beating through your chest. If you feel any pain—stop and consult your physician. Speaking of your physician, if you have a heart condition or any other physical limitation, please get his or her approval before starting any exercise program.

■

Chapter Seven

WEEKS 3 & 4: FEED YOUR BODY, NOT YOUR FAT CELLS

"YOU MEAN I can eat ice cream when I want to! I'll be part owner in Ben & Jerry's by the time I'm forty." This was Suzanne's reaction when I shared this OFF strategy. "Well, yes you can eat it, but only if you are hungry, and only if you are not overeat it. You can eat anything as long as you are feeding your body and not your fat cells."

If you truly want to feed your body instead of your fat cells:

> eat what you want
> when you are hungry
> just don't overeat it

Of course, I would love to have everyone eat a balanced, nutritious diet, but I am a firm believer in eating exactly what you want. If I told you that you could never eat chocolate again for the rest of your life, you would most likely rush to the nearest store and buy five pounds of your favorite chocolate. You always want what you can't have. I have had some clients challenge me with this philosophy. "You are a nutritionist, and you are telling me to eat truffles if I want to." I would rather have you eat a truffle every now and then, when you really want it and are hungry for it, than deprive yourself and eat twelve truffles at one sitting. Eating twelve truffles in an unconscious frenzy is a lot worse for your body and your health than choosing to eat just one truffle in moderation.

Let me share a personal story. Pizza is my favorite food in the world. In my days of deprivation, I would deny myself pizza and instead make the perfect diet meal of skinless chicken breast, cottage cheese, and carrot sticks. Later that night, I would be in and out of the kitchen grazing through the cupboards for satisfaction. Six hundred calories later and still unsatisfied, I would have a pizza delivered at midnight and eat the entire pie. Now, when I really want pizza, I have it, I don't overeat it, and I am completely and wonderfully satisfied.

You may be thinking that eating what you want means "junk food." The reason you want those foods is probably because you consider them "forbidden, bad" foods and deprive yourself. If you allow yourself to eat them, when you are hungry, and eat a moderate amount, surprise, you'll find that you don't want them as often. Just to put this in perspective, a couple of clients have related this can't have/want more phenomenon to their experience with high-protein diets. "You're absolutely right! When all I could eat was meat and eggs, all of a sudden I had an overwhelming craving for fruit." No matter what it is you can't have, you'll always want and crave it.

When Suzanne started practicing this strategy and gave herself permission to eat whatever she wanted, she ate ice cream for an entire day—breakfast, lunch, and dinner. Then ice cream took on a different meaning. It no longer meant deprivation, comfort, and ecstasy. It was simply a food choice that she could make anytime she wanted to, as long as she was hungry and she didn't overeat it. If she wanted to eat ice cream for lunch one day, she'd have it, enjoy it, and forget about it!

You will not become clinically malnourished eating ice cream or any other food for lunch. Most people feel that they have to eat the sandwich and soup first to get their nutrition, and then they can have the ice cream. Well, then you are *overeating* and will *store* the ice cream in your fat cells. If you had eaten just the ice cream and then included nutritious foods later that day, you'd have gotten your vitamins and wouldn't have stored the ice cream in your fat cells.

I'm not suggesting that you eat high fat, high sugar, nutrient-free foods all day long just because you think you want them. Good nutrition is vital. If you are truly listening to your body, it will want a variety of foods: fruits, vegetables, starch, protein—and, sometimes, fat, sugar, and salt.

If you surveyed what "naturally thin" people ate, it would be a wide variety of foods, from apples to chips and from chicken to cheeseburgers. They do not gain weight from eating these foods. The difference is whatever they eat, they eat it when they are hungry and they don't overeat it. They can walk over to the bag of chips, take a handful, and walk away. You, on the other hand, may position yourself strategically in front of the bag of chips, and stay there until the bag is empty.

The key is eating what you want without overeating when you are hungry. Easy to say and difficult to do, but maybe explaining the effect of overeating on your female fat cells will help. When you overeat, excess calories are fat-cell calories; it does not matter where they come from. They are stored in the fat cells all over your body, but particularly in the female fat cells of the hips, buttocks, and thighs. Once again, it doesn't matter what you are overeating. Any food will be stored in your fat cells if you overeat it.

Let's take apples for an in-depth explanation. Apples are a healthy choice. How can they possibly be fattening? If all your body needs to function at noon today is two apples, and

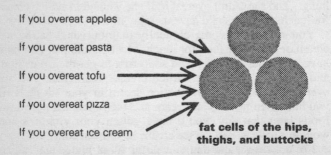

If you overeat apples

If you overeat pasta

If you overeat tofu

If you overeat pizza

If you overeat ice cream

fat cells of the hips, thighs, and buttocks

you eat six apples, the four excess apples will be converted to fat and stored as fat:

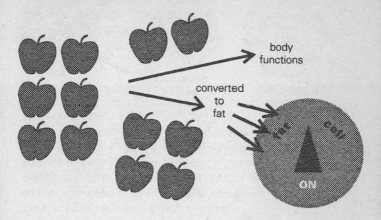

If your body needs the calories, it will use them. If your body doesn't need the calories, it will store them as fat. It could be the healthiest food in the world, but overeating it makes it a fattening food. I have a client who used to binge on cookies, cakes, pies, and ice cream. She thought if she changed her binging foods to low-fat crackers, French bread, and nonfat frozen yogurt, she would lose a lot of weight. Well, she didn't lose much weight at all because she was still overeating.

So, if undereating (as we discussed in the last chapter) and overeating feeds your fat cells, what should you do? The solution is eating moderately. When you eat moderately, your fat cells find life pretty boring and don't pay much attention. Your lipogenic enzymes are not stimulated, and your fat cells are not switched on.

But what exactly is moderate eating? There is no exact meaning, except that it is the amount of food that your body needs to function and thrive. If I told all of you to eat moderately at 1,700 calories a day, some would be overfeeding

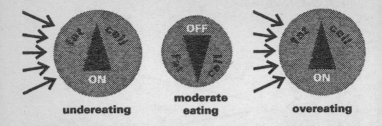

undereating   moderate   overeating
                      eating

their bodies, some would be underfeeding their bodies, and the rest would be moderately feeding their bodies. Counting calories and following a specific caloric intake does not guarantee moderate eating. Each of us has different caloric needs that can change on a daily basis. Today you might need 1,700 calories, tomorrow 1,400 calories, and the next day 2,100 calories. Stress, illness, menstruation, and other factors can influence your caloric needs. The best advice I can give you is to not deny yourself, eat when your body tells you it is hungry, and don't overeat.

You began using the **OFF** Hunger/Fullness Rating Scale in weeks 1 & 2 to identify hunger and learn how to trust your body to tell you when to eat. It is also a useful tool to identify fullness and to learn how to feed your body. It will help you to eat a moderate amount of food and prevent you from overfeeding your fat cells. I recommend keeping hunger/fullness records for a minimum of two weeks to identify what moderate eating is for you and to experience what it feels like to be "comfortable."

The OFF Hunger/Fullness Rating Scale

10 - Absolutely, positively, lie-on-the-floor stuffed
 9 - So full that you are starting to hurt
 8 - Very full and bloated

7 - Starting to feel uncomfortable
6 - Slightly overeating
5 - Perfectly comfortable
4 - First signal that your body needs food
3 - Strong signals to eat
2 - Very hungry, irritable
1 - Extreme hunger, dizziness

If you truly want to feed your body and not your fat cells, then slowly train yourself to eat moderately and *stop eating at level 5*. Every time you eat to a point above level 5, you are overeating. If you start eating at level 3 and eat to level 8, you are overeating. If you start eating at level 5, you are not hungry to begin with and your body doesn't need any calories, so anything that you eat is overeating. The typical American overeats two out of three meals a day, and usually at level 8. We are used to eating until we are "full," not until we are "comfortable." If you feel full, then you are filling your fat cells.

Laura decided that she was going to delete the word "full" from her vocabulary. In her efforts to stop eating at level 5, she found that visualization was an excellent deterrent. As she told me once, "If I want a second helping of pasta, I close my eyes and think of the next mouthful of noodles traveling down my esophagus, digesting in my stomach, being absorbed in my bloodstream, and transforming into an ugly fat globule. The lipogenic enzymes then scoop it up and slip it into a fat cell on the inside of my left thigh." Well, it's graphic, but she's a nurse and it worked for her.

There are other techniques in addition to visualization that may help you to stop at level 5, prevent overeating, and avoid turning your fat cells on. You may be a longtime member of the "Clean the Plate Club"—you may even be the president. If your goal is to always clean your plate, and you lose consciousness from the time you take the first bite until you wipe the plate clean with a piece of bread, try this:

1. Divide the food on your plate in half
2. Eat one half of it
3. Push your chair back and wait two minutes
4. Identify if you are at level 5
5. Decide if you need to eat more.
6. If you do need to eat more, divide the remainder in half and repeat the steps.

These steps have been useful with many of my clients, but as with any technique, it has to meet your needs to be successful. For Robin with her "if it's on my plate, it's in my stomach" attitude, this did not work. But she changed it a bit to fit her needs. Instead of dividing the food on her plate in half, she divided the food that she would have normally put on her plate in half. After eating the half-portion on her plate, she identified how her body felt and decided if she needed to serve herself more to be "comfortable."

If you have a difficult time leaving food on your plate, you are not alone. We have been conditioned since childhood to clean our plates. We couldn't have dessert or be excused from the table unless our plate was sparkling clean. We were constantly reminded of the starving children in the world, and today we still feel guilty about throwing food away. Whether the food ends up in your stomach or in the garbage can, it's not going to the starving children who need it.

If you eat as if you were competing for the world speed record, most likely you are overeating. When you eat quickly, your taste buds are not satisfied, and you pass right by level 5 without realizing it. Some weight-control experts recommend taking twenty to thirty minutes to eat. As Maryann interpreted it, "Great, I have thirty minutes to eat as much as I can!" Obviously, she missed the point. If you are a fast eater and think that slowing down will be helpful for you, here are a few suggestions:

- Keep your plate on the table (instead of holding the plate up to your mouth to shovel the food in).
- Cut your food into smaller pieces.

- Put your fork down between each bite.
- Chew slowly and thoroughly.
- Drink water with your meal (this will not interfere with digestion).

If you've tried these suggestions without success, make it a challenge. If you eat with someone who is a slow eater, try to take longer than they take to eat. This may be tortuous in the beginning, but it has worked for some of my clients.

Martha found that slowing down her eating in combination with the "first theory" was most helpful in determining the right amount of food for her. Supposedly, your stomach is about the size of your fist. I know it is hard to believe given the amount of food we devour at Thanksgiving and other feasts, but the stomach has amazing capabilities for expansion. Martha would match the amount of food she was about to eat with the size of her fist and found that it was the "comfortable" amount for her.

Here is a checklist of a few other techniques that may be nelpful:

- Take smaller portions (why tempt yourself).
- Use a smaller plate.
- Leave a small amount of food on your plate.
- Leave serving plates off the table.
- Sit down while eating.
- Eat only in a designated dining area.
- Don't wear elastic-waisted pants or skirt (the more you can expand, the more you may eat).
- Brush your teeth right after eating to finalize eating.

One meal of overindulgence every now and then will not sabotage your efforts. As a matter of fact, it is perfectly "normal" to overeat occasionally. Your fat cells are only turned on when you overeat on a regular basis. On Thanksgiving, you may be off the chart completely at a level 12. You haven't blown it, just focus back to level 5 at your next meal.

Some people give themselves permission to overeat if they

exercised that day. You already know that exercise releases fat from the fat cell. If you exercise today and then eat to level 9 tonight, you are only putting back what you took out. If you eat a box of crackers, and then try to exercise the calories away, you are only taking out what you put in. You'll never see a change in your body. Overeating and exercise are not a compatible pair.

This strategy of feeding your body is difficult to implement, but it is extremely important. You could be eating healthful foods, eating when you are hungry, and exercising regularly—but if you are overeating, you are always storing, and you will never permanently switch your fat cells off and outsmart them.

Now that you have all the background to Feed Your Body, Not Your Fat Cells, let's put it into practice . . .

YOUR OFF ACTION PLAN: WEEKS 3 & 4

OFF Strategy Focus: Feed Your Body, Not Your Fat Cells

OFF Goals:
1. Continue with the goals from weeks 1 & 2.
2. Learn to eat whatever you want without guilt as long as you don't overeat it.
3. Identify your fullness signals and learn to stop eating when comfortable, not full.
4. Add another day of exercise a week (or two if you are ready) and increase the duration to 20 minutes each session.

OFF Techniques:
1. Listen to your body and eat what you want.
2. Remind yourself that any food is fattening if you overeat it.

3. Use the Hunger/Fullness Scale.
4. Divide the food on your plate in half.
5. Slow down your eating.
6. Use your fist to determine a moderate amount of food.
7. Drink water with your meal.
8. Put your fork down between each bite.
9. Time your eating.
10. Chew slowly and thoroughly.
11. Take smaller portions (why tempt yourself).
12. Use a smaller plate.
13. Leave a small amount of food on your plate.
14. Leave serving plates off the table.
15. Sit down while eating.
16. Eat only in a designated dining area.
17. Don't wear elastic-waisted pants or skirt.
18. Brush your teeth right after eating.
19. **Keep food records for two weeks to practice these techniques.**

You began keeping food records in weeks 1 & 2 to identify hunger signals and to learn to eat when you are hungry. Now that you know when to start eating, it's time to learn when to stop. These strategies and food records work together in developing new skills and behaviors. Continue recording your hunger levels every hour or so, then, if you ate, record your fullness level and assess whether or not you have overeaten. Here is an example:

HUNGER/FULLNESS RECORDS FOR
FEEDING YOUR BODY

TIME	HUNGER RATING	DID YOU EAT?	FULLNESS RATING	DID YOU OVEREAT? WHY?
6:00 am	5	no		
7:00 am	4	yes	5	no
8:00 am	5	no		
9:00 am	4	no		
10:00 am	3	yes	5	no
11:00 am	5	no		
12:00 pm	4	no		
1:00 pm	3	yes	6	a little, big sandwich
2:00 pm	6	no		
3:00 pm	5	yes	7	yes, tough day
4:00 pm	6	no		
5:00 pm	5	no		
6:00 pm	4	no		
7:00 pm	3	no		
8:00 pm	2	yes	8	yes - too hungry!
9:00 pm	8	no		
10:00 pm	7	yes	8	yes - watching TV
11:00 pm	7	no		

There are many **OFF** techniques presented in this chapter to help you eat moderately to level 5, to prevent overeating, and to achieve the goal of feeding your body. Use only those techniques that make sense to you. If one technique doesn't seem to be working, move on to another one. For example, if you cannot leave food on your plate, then take smaller portions. If you cannot slow down your eating, then use your fist to determine a moderate amount of food.

I realize that keeping food records can be a tedious task, but they serve as an excellent tool to practice and assess new behaviors. There is a blank food record on the next page, but again you may find it easier to keep a small notebook with you at all times so that you can record each meal or snack. We tend to have amnesia when it comes to food, but keep in mind that fat cells have excellent memories. If you wait until the end of the day to record, will you really remember how your body felt before and after eating? Will you really remember the handful of peanuts or the second helping?

Many of my clients get frustrated at this point because they now have a second set of food records, and I still don't care what they are eating. Focusing on what to eat and what not to eat is dieting. As long as you don't overeat, you are feeding your body and outsmarting your fat cells.

YOUR NEXT STEP IN AEROBICIZING YOUR FAT CELLS

"One day of walking a week is a piece of cake, but don't worry, I didn't eat the cake while walking." Paula had a great sense of humor and enjoyed teasing me with food analogies, but she was encouraged that exercising once a week was so easy and she was ready for another day. That's what we are doing—easing exercise into your life. When you have accomplished one small exercise goal, it will be easier to accomplish the next small goal.

You've made the time and commitment to exercise once a

week for the last two weeks. *Now, it's time to fit just one more day into your schedule.*

- If you chose to ride your bike in the mornings, simply add one more morning.
- If you chose to walk at lunchtime, then block out one more lunch hour so that you will not plan to meet a friend or schedule a business luncheon.
- If you chose to go to the club on your way home from work, then bring your workout clothes one more day.

Once you've chosen your second day of exercise, you'll work on increasing the amount of time you are exercising at a moderate intensity. For the first two weeks, you did as many minutes as you could, slowly working up to 15 minutes—just add 5 more minutes to make it 20 minutes.

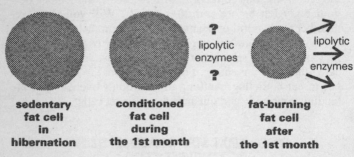

sedentary
fat cell
in
hibernation

conditioned
fat cell
during
the 1st month

fat-burning
fat cell
after
the 1st month

This first month of the OFF Plan is devoted to conditioning your fat cells to release fat. If you have not exercised for a while, your lipolytic enzymes have been in hibernation. They don't remember how to release fat. You need to wake them up, clean out the cobwebs, and give them a crash course in fat-burning. Once those lipolytic enzymes are activated after the first month, you are on your way to a leaner body.

HUNGER/FULLNESS RECORDS FOR
FEEDING YOUR BODY

TIME	HUNGER RATING	DID YOU EAT?	FULLNESS RATING	DID YOU OVEREAT? WHY?
___	___	___	___	_____
___	___	___	___	_____
___	___	___	___	_____
___	___	___	___	_____
___	___	___	___	_____
___	___	___	___	_____
___	___	___	___	_____
___	___	___	___	_____
___	___	___	___	_____
___	___	___	___	_____
___	___	___	___	_____
___	___	___	___	_____
___	___	___	___	_____
___	___	___	___	_____
___	___	___	___	_____
___	___	___	___	_____

Even if you have been exercising, you may not have conditioned fat cells and active lipolytic enzymes. You *need* to be exercising in your moderate zone to release fat and shrink your fat cells.

Remember:

- Stay in your moderate fat-burning zone.
- Sing "Old MacDonald" every 5 minutes.
- Schedule exercise on realistic days.
- If you don't like the exercise you are doing, change it!

■

Chapter Eight

WEEKS 5 & 6:
SHRINK AND
MULTIPLY YOUR MEALS

JEANIE STARTED her session one day with a confession: "I have to tell you this because I'm feeling guilty about it. I've been having a snack almost every afternoon. I know that I am not supposed to snack between meals, but I'm getting hungry at about three-thirty in the afternoon." Confession? For what? It sounds to me like everything is working perfectly. If you have been following the other OFF strategies and did not overeat lunch, your body should transmit its hunger signals at about 3:30 P.M. You need not feel guilty about snacking. You *can* and *should* eat when you are hungry. The afternoon snack will outsmart your female fat cells because it helps you to shrink and multiply your meals.

You may have already, almost unknowingly, started following this strategy as a natural progression in your behavior-change process. When you shrink your meals by eating moderately and feeding your body, you'll find that you are eating those smaller meals more frequently throughout the day. That's the beauty of the lifestyle approach to weight loss. One small, realistic change leads to another. First you start listening to your hunger signals to eat when you are hungry. Then as your body awareness grows, you start listening to your fullness signals to stop eating when comfortable. Now with both of these strategies working together, you will, naturally, start eating those smaller meals and snacks more frequently throughout the day.

For this strategy to work, we must first dispel two widely held beliefs in our society:

1. Snacking is bad.
2. Three balanced meals are good.

How many times have you been told that "snacking is bad" and causes weight gain? How many times have you been told to eat three balanced meals a day with no snacking between meals? This "snacking is a no-no" belief originated with the discovery of the candy bar and potato chips. We have equated snacking with junk food. A snack can be any food in the world. Forget the old belief that snacking is bad. Snacking between meals will cause weight gain only if you are not hungry and/or you overeat it.

With the OFF Plan, we are giving snacking a new, positive meaning. It is a way to provide a constant supply of calories to your body, and a way to prevent overeating and feeding your fat cells. Snacking is an effective tool to outsmart your female fat cells.

Now for the "three balanced meals a day is good" belief. Since grammar school, we have been taught the four-food-group approach to balanced meals. It was designed as a tool to ensure that we were getting all the vitamins and minerals important to health. Somewhere along the way, it took on the meaning that each meal should contain all four food groups. A meal must contain protein, starch, vegetable, salad, milk, and then, of course, dessert (the infamous fifth food group).

A balanced meal does not have to contain all four food groups to be healthful. As long as you get a variety of all the four food groups throughout the day (and maybe even a fifth food group thrown in every now and then), it doesn't matter when you eat them, in meals or in snacks, as far as proper nutrition goes. However, it does matter when you eat them as far as your female fat cells are concerned. The traditional meal of meat, potato, vegetable, bread, and salad is overeating—and that would be feeding your fat cells more than feeding your body.

Maybe we should think of our snacks as *mini-meals* and

our meals as *maxi-snacks*. A mini-meal or maxi-snack could be one, two, or three of the four food groups instead of all four plus dessert. It could be just the protein and vegetable or the starch and salad. It could also be all four food groups in much smaller amounts. I am not necessarily an advocate of frozen dinners, because even the "low-calorie" versions can be high in fat, but they guarantee small amounts and fit the definition of a mini-meal.

So, what have you learned about the snacking and balanced meal beliefs?

- Snacking is great when you are hungry.
- A meal can be as small as a maxi-snack.
- A snack can be as big as a mini-meal.
- Snacking doesn't have to be equated with junk food.
- A meal doesn't have to contain all four food groups.
- As long as you eat a wide variety of foods throughout the day, it doesn't matter if they are part of a meal or a snack.

Now that you have changed your snacking/meal attitude, let me convince you scientifically that shrinking and multiplying your meals is important to outsmart your female fat cells.

Let's assume you eat about 2,000 calories a day.

- If you ate the 2,000 calories in one huge 2,000-calorie meal or two large 1,000-calorie meals a day, you would be overeating and storing the excess in your female fat cells. Your body would use some of the food in those meals to function, but the majority of it would be scooped up by the lipogenic storage enzymes, and the bathroom scale would be on the rise. Eating one or two large meals also means that you are skipping meals and depriving your body for twelve to twenty-four hours. That puts you in the starvation mode. Once the fat is stored, it stays there, and you use other energy sources (such as muscle and sugar) to fuel your body.

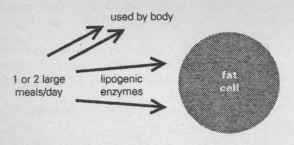

- If you ate the 2,000 calories in three balanced 666-calorie meals a day, you would be overeating a little and storing a little. You probably wouldn't gain any weight immediately, but over time, those pounds would slowly creep up on you. This is the way the typical American eats, who gains an average of three pounds a year.

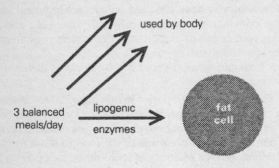

If you ate the 2,000 calories in four or five smaller 400-calorie meals a day, you would never be overeating and never be storing fat. Your body needs all the calories for immediate usage. Your fat cells would be outsmarted.

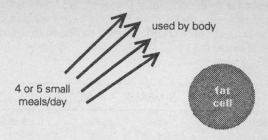

Spacing your calories out evenly throughout the day with four or five smaller meals encourages your body to burn food rather than store it. If your body needs the food, you'll burn it. If your body doesn't need it (as with overeating large meals), you'll store it. There are some who do not believe that the way you distribute calories throughout the day makes a difference. From my experience, it makes a big difference. Larger meals mean larger fat cells. Your body can use only a given amount of calories at a time to function. Therefore, your body doesn't need big meals; it needs smaller meals more frequently throughout the day.

I'm not suggesting that you eat more. I'm suggesting that you eat more often—that you take the same amount of food that you eat in two or three meals and distribute it more evenly throughout the day in four or five smaller meals.

"All right, you've convinced me that small, frequent meals will help to outsmart my female fat cells. But how do I take my two big meals a day and make them four or five smaller meals?" In small, realistic steps, just like everything else in the OFF Plan.

If you are eating one or two meals a day, I recommend that you begin eating three meals a day. By integrating three meals, you are eating a little less at those meals and storing a little less in your fat cells. Then, divide the same amount of food into four smaller meals a day. Then, eventually, if you want, divide the same food into five small meals. You have

kept your fat cells constantly guessing. Without excess calories at meals and snacks, your fat cells have switched off.

Here is a general example of how to divide the same food
into smaller meals:

	3 MEALS	4 MEALS	5 MEALS
Breakfast	cereal	cereal	cereal
	juice	juice	juice
	milk	milk	milk
Mid-morning snack			roll
			carrot sticks
Lunch	sandwich	1/2 sandwich	1/2 sandwich
	chips	chips	chips
	fruit	milk	milk
	milk		
Mid-afternoon snack		1/2 sandwich	1/2 sandwich
		fruit	fruit
Dinner	chicken	chicken	chicken
	potato	potato	potato
	carrots	carrots	salad
	salad	salad	cheesecake
	roll	roll	
	cheesecake	cheesecake	

When you are ready to start integrating four meals a day, the
mid-afternoon snack will probably work best. If you are not
overeating at lunch, you will probably be hungry by 3:30 or
4:00 P.M. Most people wait until they get home from work to
eat. They are starving, make a dash for the kitchen, and eat
standing in front of the sink in an unconscious frenzy. The mid-
afternoon snack will prevent you from being overhungry at

dinner. Many of my clients who eat sandwiches for lunch find that saving half of the sandwich for the afternoon snack is easiest. If you have skipped your afternoon snack for one reason or another, then have a roll or some crackers when you get home to take the edge off and bring you back to consciousness.

Planning ahead for accessible snacks is essential for this strategy to work. Whether it be in your desk drawer, the glove compartment, or in your purse, keep some pretzels, crackers, fruit, or other snacks that you like. If you are an "if it's there, I'll eat it" person, you may not want to make snacks too accessible. Instead, when you are hungry, go to the cafeteria or store to get it.

You may already be having a snack at around 3:30 P.M. to beat the mid-afternoon slump, but what is it? "Well, usually a candy bar, but it can be anything with sugar to give me a quick pick-me-up." A candy bar may give you a short burst of energy, but the result is an all-time energy low. Think of your mid-afternoon snacks as being power snacks. There are two different power snacks depending on your needs. *Starches* are the best power snack choice for physical energy. Starches give your muscles energy for exercise. If you work out before dinner, some crackers, pretzels, or a piece of bread will give you a physical energy boost. *Protein* is the best power snack for brain concentration. (I know you think of protein for muscle; it may build muscle, but it doesn't provide energy to your muscles.) For your brain, protein may be converted to powerful brain chemicals that increase your alertness and concentration. If you have an important meeting, or a test, or a deadline to meet, having a protein power snack may help you feel more productive, less stressed, and less fatigued. Here are some examples of protein power snacks: half of a roast beef or turkey sandwich, a chicken breast, nonfat yogurt, or cottage cheese.

I have strongly recommended eating four or five times a day with maxi-snacks and mini-meals, but some women claim that they are not overeating breakfast and are not hungry in the morning, or they are not overeating lunch and are not hungry in the afternoon. If that is the case, don't eat mid-morning or mid-afternoon—listen to your body.

If you are not feeling hungry more often, then ask yourself, "Am I still overeating?" You may be eating considerably less at meals, and you may not feel uncomfortably stuffed anymore, but you still may be overeating past the point of being perfectly comfortable. We are so used to eating large meals and feeling full that it has clouded our perception of how our bodies really feel after eating. Using the Hunger/Fullness Rating Chart, assess how you feel after eating and ask, "Am I still overeating?"

10
  9 ← how much you used to eat
  8
  7 ← you are eating less, but you're still overeating
  6
  5 ← this is not overeating, it's 100% comfortable
  4
  3
  2
  1

How can you be sure that you are not overeating? The answer lies partly in how soon you get hungry again. To be confident that you are truly not overeating and are taking in the moderate amount of calories that your body needs, your body should tell you it's hungry in another three to four hours. It takes about three to four hours to digest and use a moderate amount of food and about six hours to digest and store a large amount of food.

Based on my experience with helping women to shrink and multiply their meals, the barriers and concerns that you may be dealing with are:

• Fear of weight gain.
• Lack of consistency during the weekends.
• No time or opportunity to eat more often.

"If I give myself permission to eat more frequently, my life will be one big binge and I'll **gain weight.**" No you won't. If you have followed the previous strategies and have taken it slowly and realistically, you are fully prepared to listen to your body, eat when you are hungry, eat a moderate amount, and distribute your calories more evenly throughout the day. The diet mentality has led us to believe that we should skip meals and eat less often to lose weight. The opposite is true: Eating smaller amounts more often is the secret to weight loss.

Some experts believe that our bodies were biologically designed to eat smaller, more frequent meals. If young children were left to their own eating instincts, they probably would never eat a meal but instead would snack periodically throughout the day. As concerned parents, we force them to sit down to meals and go against their natural eating instincts. Perhaps we should all eat more like children, and let our children follow their natural eating behaviors.

Many people who are currently at a more comfortable weight got there by eating this way. "Martha baffles me. She's lost weight, is a size eight, and eats all day long. If I ate like she eats, I'd weigh more than three Marthas put together." That's your perception, but, in reality, most of the Marthas of the world eat small amounts frequently throughout the day. They eat a handful here, a small plate there—not the whole bag, box, or container. That's the difference. They don't eat a lot all day long, they eat a little all day long.

I know you are thinking of some thin people who eat large amounts frequently throughout the day. They are *not* reading this book, but a few do exist. Some people are born lucky when it comes to their metabolism and weight. Some day it may catch up with them as their metabolism slows with age, but, until then, they are the exception to the rule.

Some clients may be fearful of this strategy, but there is a difference between people who eat more often because they are eating smaller meals and are hungry more often and others who:

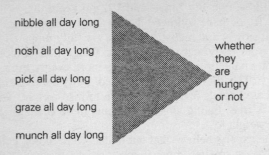

nibble all day long

nosh all day long

pick all day long

graze all day long

munch all day long

whether
they
are
hungry
or not

Whatever word you use, whether you nibble, nosh, pick, munch, or graze, if you are not hungry, your body doesn't need those calories and you will store them in your female fat cells.

Some women find it easy to eat small, frequent meals during the week, but have difficulty during the **weekend.** It's Saturday and you have plans to go to dinner with friends. You slept a little later and you had a late breakfast and are not hungry again until 3:00 P.M. So you say to yourself, "I'm going out to that wonderful Italian restaurant tonight. I'd better not eat lunch. It's too late anyway, and I don't want to spoil my appetite. I'll save up my calories so I can eat more fettuccine and garlic bread tonight." The only thing you will be saving is more fat in your fat cells. You get seated at the restaurant at 8:00 P.M. You are absolutely starving, go crazy on the bread, order an appetizer, and eat your entire plate of fettuccine to get your money's worth. If you had eaten at 3:00 P.M., when you were hungry, you could have prevented overeating at the restaurant.

Even if you are not fearful of weight gain and can be consistent during weekends, you may find **time constraints** a barrier to small frequent meals. Margarite had a job that gave no breaks, and she could not eat at her desk. She thought that eating less more often would be impossible for her to implement given her lifestyle. She could not eat a morning or afternoon snack. The only thing that was realistic for her was to keep some crackers in the glove compartment of her car and eat a couple during her commute home. Analyze your daily schedule and discover what is feasible for you.

Perhaps the many other extended benefits of small, frequent meals will help you to overcome the barriers to this strategy:

- You'll have more energy.
- You'll control your PMS symptoms.
- You'll manage stress better.

"I have **more energy** now than I have ever had in my life." I hear this over and over again. There are two reasons why you have (or will soon have) increased vitality and energy. First, you are no longer overeating. When you overeat, your stomach gets the majority of your blood supply for the lengthy digestive process. Blood is directed away from your brain and to your stomach. Without the blood, oxygen, and nutrients, your brain starts to wind down and you start feeling sleepy. Ever wonder why you are so tired after a large Sunday meal? Ever wonder why you are compelled to take a nap after your Thanksgiving meal?

The second reason for a boost in overall energy has to do with the effects on blood sugar levels. When blood sugar levels are either significantly above or below normal, you are

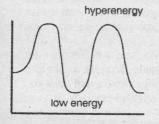

2 meals a day

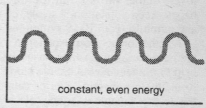

5 meals a day

not at your best. With high blood sugar levels, your brain is getting too much sugar, and you have excitable, unproductive energy. With low blood sugar levels, your brain is not getting enough sugar, and you have low, sluggish energy. Eating small, frequent meals results in a more stable blood sugar level, and a higher, more consistent level of energy.

For women who experience **premenstrual changes,** small, frequent meals may make your monthly hormonal and emotional fluctuations more tolerable and controllable. Like the majority of most premenopausal women, I also experience PMS. Some months are worse than others, but I have found that eating small, frequent meals makes a big difference. It helps so much that on those worst months, my husband, Paul, reminds me to eat more frequently. He has also given a new definition to PMS: To him it doesn't mean premenstrual syndrome, it means "*Paul Must Suffer.*" And, you know, as much as I hate to admit it—sometimes he's right.

A week or so before your period, you may be more sensitive to fluctuations in your blood sugar. When more than four hours has passed since your last meal, blood sugar levels drop below normal, and the symptoms of PMS intensify. You get irritable, moody, and sensitive. Your protesting brain says, "Give me sugar—NOW." This may be one of the reasons why women crave more sugar and go on uncontrollable sugar (usually chocolate) binges a few days before their periods. By eating small frequent meals, and keeping your blood sugar levels stable throughout the day, you'll keep your brain happy, keep your moods stable, control your sugar cravings, and minimize your PMS symptoms.

Whether or not you experience PMS, and whether you are premenopausal or postmenopausal, small, frequent meals also help to **manage stress.** Stable blood sugar levels will help you to maintain a certain level of calmness and stability in your day-to-day struggle of trying to achieve more and more in less and less time. When blood sugar levels are either too high or too low, your physiology is more stressed, and you become more emotionally stressed. When blood sugar levels are stable, your brain and physiology are more stable and less stressed.

In addition to eating smaller, more frequent meals, there are many relaxation and coping techniques to help reduce stress—and I encourage you to use them on a regular basis. Women are under more stress than ever before in history. There is the constant pressure to "act like women, think like men, and work like dogs." I don't remember who said this, but I wish I had.

Now that you have all the background to shrink and multiply your meals, let's put this strategy into practice . . .

YOUR <u>OFF</u> ACTION PLAN: WEEKS 5 & 6

OFF Strategy Focus: Shrink and Multiply Your Meals

OFF Goals:
1. Continue with goals from weeks 1–4.
2. Learn to eat and enjoy smaller, more frequent meals throughout the day.
3. Plan your day with mini-meals and maxi-snacks.
4. Add one more day of exercise and increase the duration to 30 minutes each session.

OFF Techniques:
1. Analyze your beliefs about snacking.
2. Analyze your beliefs about balanced meals.
3. Think of your meals as maxi-snacks.
4. Think of your snacks as mini-meals.
5. Make a list of mini-meals and maxi-snacks.
6. Eat 1, 2, or 3 of the food groups instead of all 4 plus dessert.

7. Keep snacks in accessible places: desk, car, briefcase.

8. Eat a power snack for the 3:30 P.M. slump: starch for your workout or protein for your concentration.

9. Divide your lunch in half and eat the second half for the afternoon snack.

10. Keep blood sugar levels stable for maximum energy.

11. Keep blood sugar levels stable to manage stress.

12. Keep blood sugar levels stable to control PMS.

13. Use the Hunger/Fullness Rating Scale to make sure that you are not overeating.

14. **Keep food records for two weeks to practice these techniques.**

I know—yuck—more food records. These are slightly different. You are already recording your hunger and fullness level, so that part is easy. Now I am going to ask you to record the times when you are eating your meals or snacks and the approximate amounts. I'm finally asking you to write down what you are eating, but I really don't care what it is, just *how* you are distributing what you are eating throughout the day.

You may find that some days you are hungry five times and other days only three or even just two times during the day. It's most important to stay in tune with your body and eat when you are hungry. Don't force yourself to eat if you are not hungry.

Keep records of small, frequent meals for at least two weeks. On the following pages are an example and a blank food record for you to use as a guideline.

YOUR NEXT STEP IN AEROBICIZING
YOUR FAT CELLS

Congratulations!! You've made it through the first month of exercise. I'm congratulating you because most people stop exercising within the first month for three reasons:

1. They chose the wrong exercise and didn't like it.
2. They chose the wrong time and couldn't keep the commitment.
3. They overexercised and the pain and exhaustion just wasn't worth it.

You chose the right exercise, the right time of day, and the right intensity by exercising moderately. You're exercising twice a week 20 minutes each time. Now, add one more day and 10 minutes to your exercise sessions. By the end of week 6 you'll be exercising three times a week for 30 minutes each session.

If you have any doubt as to whether you've chosen the right exercise, try another activity to make it more pleasurable. If you are using the stationary bike and find it to be the most boring thing you've ever done in your life, don't torture yourself. You'll come up with a million excuses not to place your buttocks on the seat.

HUNGER/FULLNESS RECORD FOR SHRINKING AND MULTIPLYING YOUR MEALS

MEAL/ SNACK	TIME	HUNGER LEVEL	APPROXIMATE AMOUNTS	FULLNESS LEVEL
breakfast	6:30am	4	1 c cereal	5
			1 c milk	
			6 oz juice	
snack	9:30am	4	1/2 c yogurt	5
			1 pear	
lunch	12:15pm	3	1/2 sandwich	5
			1 apple	
			1 soft drink	
snack	4:30pm	3	1/2 sandwich	5
			1 cookie	
dinner	7:45pm	3	4 oz meat	5
			1 c carrots	
			1/2 c rice	

HUNGER/FULLNESS RECORD FOR SHRINKING AND MULTIPLYING YOUR MEALS

MEAL/ SNACK	TIME	HUNGER LEVEL	APPROXIMATE AMOUNTS	FULLNESS LEVEL
___	___	___	___	___
			___	
			___	
			___	
___	___	___	___	___
			___	
			___	
			___	
___	___	___	___	___
			___	
			___	
			___	
___	___	___	___	___
			___	
			___	
			___	
___	___	___	___	___
			___	
			___	
			___	

This is a very important next step in your exercise program. It is the start of your fat-burning exercise program. Up until now, you have conditioned your fat cells to release fat Now, you are entering the "fat burning zone." You now have all the ingredients to use oxygen (O_2) and the lipolytic enzymes to release fat from your fat cells:

$$O_2 + \text{lipolytic enzymes} + 30 \text{ minutes} = \text{fat release}$$

Each time you exercise for 30 minutes, you are starting to release fat. You will be starting to shrink your fat cells three times a week. Hooray!! I do have some suggestions for those three days to maximize the benefits. Spread the three days throughout the week. If you exercise Monday, Tuesday, and Wednesday—and then not again until the next Monday— you will not get as much benefit than if you separated the days. At least separate the third day—do it Monday, Tuesday, and Friday. You've probably heard that exercising every other day is best, and, ideally, it is. But ideal may not be what is realistic for you, so find what is right for you.

Exercise is not cumulative. The 30 minutes must be done all at once. Exercising in the morning for 15 minutes and in the evening for 15 minutes adds up to 30 minutes—but you won't be using fat energy. You get started . . . then stop. You start activating the lipolytic enzymes . . . then stop. Thirty *consecutive* minutes is necessary to activate your lipolytic enzymes and begin shrinking your fat cells. Every time you get the urge to cut your exercise session short, visualize this graph.

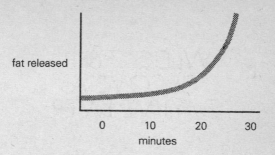

Remember:

- Stay in your moderate fat-burning zone.
- Sing "Old MacDonald" every 5 minutes.
- Schedule exercise on realistic days.
- If you don't like the exercise you are doing, change it!!

Chapter Nine

■

WEEKS 7 & 8. BECOME A DAYTIME EATER

❝ AM doing a terrific job during the day. I'm eating when I am hungry, I'm not overeating lunch, and I'm having a mid-afternoon snack—but at night, it's another story. As soon as I get home from work, it's like I'm a different person. I eat continuously from six to eleven. During the day, I feel in complete control. At night, I feel completely out of control."

If you are feeling like you transform from a Dr. Jekyll to a Mr. Hyde when the sun starts to set, then this chapter will be vital to your success on the OFF Plan. Most people find i* much easier to control their eating behavior during the day. You're busy, you may be away from home, you're not around food. At night, you're home, you're around food, you're thinking about food, commercials remind you of food, and the kitchen is always right around the corner.

Are you a nocturnal eater? Most likely the answer is a strong yes. The typical American eats about 70 percent of her calories after five o'clock at night—and the typical American is overweight. As a matter of fact, it may be the underlying explanation of why we are an overweight society. Here's the reason: Your metabolism and caloric needs are lower at night than at any other time during the day. Your metabolism is fastest in the morning and afternoon, then begins to slow down, with the lowest level at night. When your metabolism is low, your fat cells are most active. So, at night, when your metabolism is low and your caloric intake is high, you are more likely to turn fat cells on for storage and gain weight.

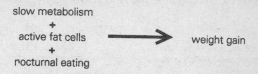

slow metabolism
+
active fat cells ⟶ weight gain
+
nocturnal eating

"You mean my fat cells awaken when my body starts to fall asleep? Don't fat cells ever sleep?" Unlike the rest of your body, your fat cells do not require slumber. As you enter dreamland, your fat cells seize the opportunity for storage. As you are dreaming of sugar plums, your fat cells are storing them.

As the sun sets, the lipogenic storage enzymes become more active. If you are a nocturnal eater, more calories are going to be stored than utilized by your body. You will feed your fat cells, not your body—even if your total calorie intake is not excessive.

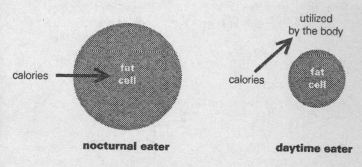

nocturnal eater　　　　　　**daytime eater**

My goal is to help you "match your eating to your metabolism"—so that you eat the majority of your small, frequent meals when your metabolism is highest, which is during the first twelve hours of the day. If you wake up at 6:00 A.M. and your body needs about 2,000 calories a day to function (to make the calculations easy), it will burn about 75 percent of those calories (or 1,500 calories) from 6:00 A.M. to 6:00 P.M. and only about 25 percent of those calories (or 500 calories) from 6:00 P.M. to 6:00 A.M. the next morning.

	BODY'S CALORIC NEEDS
6:00 A.M. to 6:00 P.M.	1,500 calories
6:00 P.M. to 6:00 A.M.	500 calories

Most likely, your eating is the reverse of what your body needs. You wake up in the morning and have a muffin and coffee, if anything at all. You are watching your calories, so you have a salad with low-calorie dressing for lunch. You get home from work at 6:00 P.M. and go directly into the kitchen for some cheese and crackers, you nibble a bit on what you are preparing for dinner, you eat the dinner, and then you wander into the kitchen for at least two snacks during your TV/relaxation time.

6:00 A.M. to 6:00 P.M.	6:00 P.M. to 6:00 A.M.
muffin and coffee	cheese and crackers
salad with lo-cal dressing	hunk of bread
	couple of carrot sticks
	dinner—chicken
	rice
	carrots
	salad
	bread
	popcorn
	frozen yogurt

From 6:00 A.M.. to 6:00 P.M.: Your metabolism is working overtime. It wants to burn a lot of calories for your body to function, but you gave it only a few calories. Oh, well—your loss. You could have eaten more and burned more.

From 6:00 P.M. to 6:00 A.M.: Your metabolism has punched the clock—work is over. It's done burning and is preparing for rest. This is when your fat cells report to work. The calorie-burning is over—it's calorie-storage time, and you gave it plenty of calories to store.

	YOUR BODY NEEDED	YOU ATE	DIFFERENCE
6 A.M. to 6 P.M.	1,500 calories	500 calories	-1,000 calories
6 P.M. to 6 A.M.	500 calories	1,500 calories	+1,000 calories

The above is a general example, and your body may work a bit differently, but if you eat in a similar way, every night there is a calorie excess. It may not be a 1,000-calorie excess as in the above situation, it may be a 200- or a 500- or an 800-calorie excess, but it *is* an excess. Where do these extra calories go? Directly to the fat cells of your buttocks, hips, and thighs. Each night, you will not be an eyewitness to your fat cells growing, but, over time, the hips will spread, the buttocks will bulge, and the thighs will expand.

One of my more challenging clients, Marypat, thought that she had me in a corner: "Now wait a minute, I may be eating 1,000 calories too many a night—but I'm eating 1,000 calories too few during the day. I'll just use what I store from the night before." No you won't. Whenever you take in fewer calories than your body needs, you're putting your body into a semistarvation state. Remember what we talked about with dieting: A calorie deficit causes fat protection. Your body uses sugar and protein stores for needed calories, not fat. What really happens is that you store 1,000 calories as fat at night, and take 1,000 calories from your muscle mass and sugar stores during the day. You can't starve a fat cell.

The solution is quite simple: *Match your eating to your metabolism.* Become a daytime eater by eating more of your food during the day and less at night. Daytime calories will be burned; nighttime calories will be stored. It is that simple.

There are two effective ways to become a daytime eater and match your eating to your metabolism:

1. Eat your dinner earlier.
2. Make your dinner smaller.

There was a physician in the 1930s who put his patients on a "new, guaranteed weight-loss diet." All of his patients who followed this diet lost weight and kept it off for the rest of their lives. Can you imagine what his diet consisted of? The dead giveaway is that it worked, so it really wasn't a diet at all. The only recommendation was to eat dinner by 5:00 P.M. He didn't restrict foods, count calories, or push packaged foods. Whatever his clients were eating, they just had to eat it by 5:00 P.M. Having an early dinner has proved successful for over fifty years, but, unfortunately, our schedules today do not permit five o'clock dinners. But how early could you eat dinner? Could you eat at 6:30 instead of 7:30? Could you eat an early dinner on Sundays? Every little change makes a difference.

If you cannot eat dinner earlier, by about 5:00 or 6:00, because you work late or have other commitments, then make your dinner meal as small as possible. If you have been eating small, frequent meals from the previous strategy, I hope you have found that the mid-afternoon snack has already helped you to eat a smaller dinner. It certainly helped Jeanette. When she began bringing pretzels to work for her 3:30 P.M. snack, she soon discovered that she no longer needed to eat when she walked in the door at night. We planned her walk right after work so that she didn't have a chance to think about food, and right after her smaller dinner, she brushed her teeth. When she got tired, instead of eating, she went to bed. She became a daytime eater, lost sixteen pounds of fat, and outsmarted her fat cells.

Eat a reasonable lunch, have a mid-afternoon snack, and think of your dinner as an evening snack. A bowl of cereal, soup, a salad, half a sandwich, or yogurt and fruit can be a satisfying dinner. Have you ever thought of having a bowl of cereal for dinner? Your dinner may still be the largest meal of the day compared to your other mini-meals and maxi-snacks—but you still want it to be as small as possible. And, remember, you also want to make it as early as possible.

The large, late dinner meal is a product of American society. We eat a small breakfast (if any at all), a moderate lunch, and a big dinner. This is directly opposite to our metabolic needs. Most other cultures eat their largest meal midday. It is no surprise that these cultures do not have the weight problem we do. They burn instead of store. This is not an ingenious strategy that I made up to outsmart your female fat cells. This is the way your European friends and relatives eat, and this is the way your grandparents and ancestors used to eat. Lunch used to be called "dinner," and dinner used to be called "supper." Supper was their smallest meal of the day. As the dinner meal became larger, we became larger people.

With industrialization and the nine-to-five job, we no longer have time for a big breakfast and lunch. We rush to get to work on time and we have a "lunch hour" where we are lucky to get thirty minutes. We are away from our families all day long, and dinner has become our largest, family-oriented, social meal. You do not have to lose this special time with family and friends. Does a dinner have to be huge to be social? Why not have the focus be on pleasurable conversation instead of eating?

"I want to make my dinner smaller and earlier, but what about my family?" A smaller, earlier dinner is appropriate for the entire family. If you analyze young children's natural eating behavior, they would much rather snack than eat a meal and, if given the chance, would skip dinner altogether. Could it be that our bodies are biologically programmed to eat small meals, with the majority of the food consumed during the day?

Even though this strategy is appropriate for the entire family, you may get some very strong resistance if you try to change their behavior. "Honey, I shrunk the dinner." Your partner, husband, children, or whomever you eat dinner with may not be happy when they sit down to dinner and find it has shrunk to half its original size. The last thing I want to do is to create family chaos. You can explain to them the benefit of a smaller dinner, you can have them read this chapter, but they may not be ready or may not want to change. You cannot change anyone else's behavior, but you can change your own. Sit down with them, serve them bigger portions, and serve yourself smaller ones.

So far, there have been two parts to this strategy:

1. Make your dinner as early as possible.
2. Make your dinner as small as possible.

But what about after dinner? That's the important third part:

3. Learn to control your nighttime snacking.

Margie was eating dinner by 6:00 P.M., and it was about half the size it used to be. That was the easy part. The hard part was what went on after dinner. She would snack continuously from eight to ten at night. Nighttime nibbling is a guaranteed fat-cell enlarger. Your metabolism is winding down from the day, and you are definitely not hungry because you've recently eaten dinner. The later at night you eat, the more of it will be stored in your fat cells.

Nighttime snacking is an American pastime. We are home at night, we are around food, we are reminded of food with commercials, and we use food for comfort. Here are some of the reasons my clients give for needing to snack at night:

My partner-in-crime made me do it. Your husband, partner, or roommate may be your partner-in-crime. "Do you want some ice cream?" they innocently ask, or maybe they don't even ask and just bring you a heaping bowl of your favorite flavor. It may help them to feel less guilty because there is safety in numbers. You may have been having ice cream together every night at nine for the past ten years—but that doesn't mean that you have to do it for the next ten years. Talk to your eating partner-in-crime. Ask him or her to refrain from offering you food, or, if necessary, request that the ice cream be eaten in another room.

Food talks to me at night. Becky claimed that certain foods had vocal cords. "Becky, this is your favorite ice cream bar calling. I'm in the freezer underneath the low-calorie frozen dinner. Come and get me." If this happens to you, and you can't keep food in the house without it torturing you with temptation—don't keep it in the house. But I don't want you to deprive yourself, either. If you really want it, go down to the store and get it. For you to get in the car and drive to get it, you'll have to really want it.

Food helps me fall asleep. Some people claim insomnia if they do not have a bedtime snack: "I can't sleep unless I eat something right before bed." What do you eat? "A double decker ham and swiss on rye." Your fat cells are going to love that snack—it's a meal. It is true that when your stomach is full, you get sleepy. Your blood supply is directed away from your brain and toward your stomach for digestion. It may make you sleepy, but it also makes you fat. I'm not asking you to go to bed hungry. You are supposed to eat when you are hungry, but are you really hungry for the sandwich? When was the last time you tried going to bed without the sandwich? If it was about three years ago, try again. If you really are hungry before bedtime, have a couple of crackers or a glass of milk.

Food helps me to relax. You've been up since 5:30 A.M. so that you would have time for your morning aerobic walk. You got ready for work, got your two children dressed, and dropped them off at day-care. You missed your car-pool ride, got stuck in traffic, and arrived late for your morning meeting. Your secretary called in sick, your mother-in-law called, and you had twelve phone calls to return. You had to meet a deadline before noon, meet a client for lunch, and meet two other deadlines by five. You picked up the dry cleaning, picked up your kids from day-care, and prepared dinner. You cleaned up the kitchen, gave the kids a bath, and your mother-in-law called again. HELP!!! No wonder some women use food to help them wind down from the day's stress. But does it really help? It usually results in more stress because you feel guilty afterward.

Whatever your reasons for snacking at night—does it really give you what you need? The best advice I was ever given was by my co-worker, Dr. Dee Tivenan, who is a terrific therapist. She has helped me and many of my clients to get in the habit of asking ourselves:

1. What am I feeling?
2. What do I really need?

Two very simple questions that uncover often complex, but very useful, answers. Most people are not in touch with their feelings, and if you don't know what you are really feeling, you don't know what you really need. Sometimes we use food so that we won't feel. You'll continue to snack at night until you identify what you are feeling and what you really need. The more you get in the habit of asking yourself these questions, the more you will discover that food is not at all what you need.

Here are a few examples of what you may really need to deal with your feelings:

What are you feeling?	What do you really need?
Tired?	To go to bed? To relax with a book?
Stressed?	Deep breathing? A walk?
Lonely?	To call a friend? To go to a movie?
Depressed?	A hug? A bouquet of flowers?
Angry?	To scream? To punch a pillow?

What you personally need may be different from the above examples, but you won't know until you ask the questions. You need to get into the habit of asking yourself what you really need at that moment. "I'd be done with the package of cookies before I'd remember that I forgot to ask the questions." Bonnie had to put reminders on the cupboards and refrigerator to help her get into the habit.

One more point to mention about nighttime snacking. It gets your body completely out of sync. If you snack at night, you are not hungry in the morning, so you skip breakfast. Then, you don't start consuming your day's calories until noon when you are starving, you get a big dinner, then snack again that night. When a client strongly states, "I am never hungry in the morning, the mere thought of food makes me nauseous," I quickly ask about her nighttime nibbling. If you eat at night, very little digestion occurs during sleep, you wake up with a full stomach, so of course you are not going to feel hungry. As soon as you start matching your eating to your metabolism and eat less at night, you'll find that you are hungry in the morning and want to eat.

You may deviate from the norm with your metabolism. Some people are night owls. They have a higher level of energy in the evening, stay up until 3:00 A.M. and sleep until 10:00 A.M. Make this strategy work for you by matching your eating to your personal metabolism. Focus on eating during the first twelve hours of your day, no matter what time you wake up. If you work nights, you'll have to arrange this a bit differently and have your biggest meal when you wake up and before going to work.

Now that you have all the background to become a daytime eater, let's put this strategy into practice . . .

YOUR OFF ACTION PLAN: WEEKS 7 & 8

OFF Strategy Focus: Become a Daytime Eater

OFF Goals:
1. Continue with goals from weeks 1–6.
2. Match your eating to your metabolism by consuming more of your calories during the day and fewer at night.
3. Learn to control your nighttime snacking.
4. Exercise three times a week (if you get the urge for a fourth day, go for it), and increase the duration to 35 minutes each session.

OFF Techniques:
1. Eat your dinner meal as early as possible.
2. Make your dinner meal as small as possible.

3. Think of your lunch as dinner.
4. Think of your dinner as supper.
5. Think of your dinner meal as your evening snack.
6. Include an afternoon snack so that you will not be overhungry at dinner.
7. Keep busy after dinner.
8. Use other strategies to help you relax.
9. Use other strategies to help you sleep.
10. Remind yourself that fat cells never sleep.
11. Ask yourself, "Am I really hungry?"
12. Ask yourself, "What am I really feeling? What do I really need?"
13. Make a list of other activities (besides eating) that will give you what you really need.
14. Exercise in the evening.
15. Use 6:00 P.M. as your marker for a slower metabolism.
16. If you work the night shift, have your largest meal when you wake up and before work.
17. Use the Hunger/Fullness Rating Scale.
18. **Keep food records for two weeks to practice these techniques.**

Obviously, record keeping is an integral part of the <u>OFF</u> Plan. Each two-week segment adds on new skills and positive behaviors. This set of food records focuses on the *timing* of your small meals and snacks (still not your food choices) to encourage you to become a daytime eater. You'll still record your hunger and fullness levels and how you are distributing your meals and snacks. The additional emphasis will be on the time of day you are eating. Here is an example:

HUNGER/FULLNESS RECORDS FOR
DAYTIME EATING

TIME	MEAL OR SNACK	HUNGER LEVEL	APPROX-IMATE AMOUNTS	FULL-NESS LEVEL
6:30am	breakfast	4	1 c cereal 1 c milk 6 oz juice	5
9:30am	snack	4	½ c yogurt 1 fruit	5
12:15pm	lunch	3	½ sandwich 1 fruit 1 soft drink	5
3:00pm	snack	4	½ sandwich	5
6:00pm	dinner	3	3 oz meat 1 c carrots ½ c rice	5

What time did you wake up? *6:00 am*
Did you eat most of your small, frequent meals in the first twelve hours of the day? *Yes! Even ate dinner by 6 pm.!*

As with each of the previous strategies, choose only those techniques that are realistic for you. If you don't get home from work until 7:30, it will be impossible to eat an early dinner. But you can have a late afternoon snack and a smaller dinner.

This strategy makes complete sense (I hope you agree), but you may be feeling a bit frustrated.

- How can I eat more during the day when my job is so stressful, I don't even have time to go to the bathroom?
- How can I eat a bigger breakfast when I have to get two kids ready for school?
- How can I have a bigger lunch when I have a thirty-minute lunch break and often have to run around doing errands?

Maybe you can't, but the question is not what you *can't* do—it's what you *can* do.

- Can I make my dinner meal a little earlier?
- Can I make my dinner meal a little smaller?
- Can I eat a mid-morning snack?
- Can I eat a mid-afternoon snack?
- Can I get out of the bedtime snack habit?

You do not have to follow this strategy every day for the rest of your life. If you go out to a late dinner this weekend with friends, so what? Eating a larger meal late at night every now and then will not result in bigger fat cells. Eating a large meal late at night every night will result in bigger fat cells.

Keep food records for the next two weeks. On the following page is a blank food record for you to use as a guideline.

HUNGER/FULLNESS RECORDS FOR DAYTIME EATING

TIME	MEAL OR SNACK	HUNGER LEVEL	APPROX-IMATE AMOUNTS	FULLNESS LEVEL
____	____	____	____	____
			____	
			____	
____	____	____	____	____
			____	
			____	
____	____	____	____	____
			____	
			____	
____	____	____	____	____
			____	
			____	
____	____	____	____	____
			____	
			____	

What time did you wake up?
Did you eat most of your small, frequent meals in the first twelve hours of the day?

YOUR NEXT STEP IN AEROBICIZING YOUR FAT CELLS

At this point, every extra minute you spend exercising at the fat-releasing moderate intensity will be an additional fat-burning minute. After 30 minutes, your lipolytic enzymes are activated and prepared to release fat.

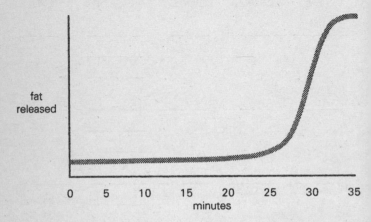

During this next two-week segment, add 5 minutes to your workouts. By the end of the two weeks, you will be exercising three times a week for 35 minutes each session. That's the minimum you have to do, but you are not limited to the minimum. If you are feeling fit and energetic, keep going for 40 or 45 minutes. If you want, you can even add a fourth day for 35 minutes.

Remember:

• Stay in your moderate fat-burning zone.
• Sing "Old MacDonald."
• Schedule exercise on realistic days.

■

Chapter Ten

WEEKS 9 & 10 FAT-PROOF YOUR DIET

"WELL, IT'S about time. This is the last **OFF** strategy, and you are finally going to tell me what I can and can't eat." No I'm not. I'm going to give you a wealth of information about fat and the fat content of foods so that *you* can make well-informed decisions about what *you* put into your body.

I've said it a hundred time in this book ... and I'm going to say it again: No food will cause weight gain as long as you eat it when you are hungry and you don't overeat it. And any food will cause weight gain if you eat it when you are not hungry and your overeat it.

Now that I've said that again, I must take it one step further: If we rate foods based on their likelihood of becoming stored fat in your fat cells, high-fat foods would be number one. When you overeat them, they are more fattening than high carbohydrate and high protein foods. The reason: Fat is already in its storage form. It is hassle-free and effortless for your fat cells to take the fat that you just ate in the cheeseburger and fries and store it.

Carbohydrates and protein would tie for second place. They require energy and effort to convert them to fat before they can be stored as fat. So, when you overeat, it makes sense that fat is more fattening than carbohydrates and protein. How much more fattening? Read on.

If you eat an extra 100 calories of fat that your body

doesn't need, it takes only about 3 calories to digest and metabolize the fat. You will find 97 of those fat calories stored in your fat cell:

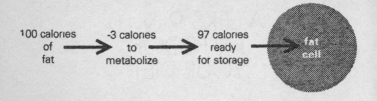

100 calories of fat ➝ -3 calories to metabolize ➝ 97 calories ready for storage ➝ fat cell

If you eat an extra 100 calories of carbohydrates or protein that your body doesn't need, it takes at least 25 calories to digest and convert them to fat. You will find 75 of those calories stored in your thighs:

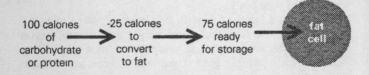

100 calories of carbohydrate or protein ➝ -25 calories to convert to fat ➝ 75 calories ready for storage ➝ fat cell

"So what you are telling me is that if I am going to binge, I'm better off wolfing down a French baguette or an entire turkey than a bag of potato chips." Laura was looking for a way to binge and lose weight simultaneously. Sorry, there is no way. You'll still gain weight binging on that baguette; you'll just gain a little more weight binging on the potato chips.

Overeating any food will lead to larger fat cells, but overeating fat will lead to the largest fat cell of all—about 25 percent larger than carbohydrates and protein. That's the first reason to reduce your fat intake. When there's a first, it's always followed by a second. Here's the second reason: Fat is not the preferred energy source for your body to function at it's most efficient capacity. Carbohydrates are the preferred energy source for all of your organs and cells (except your fat cells because they don't require energy). The majority of the public still believes that carbohydrates (often called starches) are fattening. Breads, potato, pasta, rice, and all the other starches are not fattening if you don't overeat them. It's the fat we put on them that makes them fattening—the butter, margarine, sour cream, and cream cheese.

Carbohydrates are digested and absorbed as glucose, which is the best energy source for all cells and all organs. If you eat a potato, it will become glucose in your bloodstream, travel through the capillaries, and enter into brain (or liver or lung) cells to be utilized.

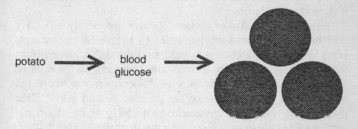

potato ⟶ blood glucose ⟶

preferred energy source for your body's cells

Protein is not the preferred energy source for your cells (as we discussed in Chapter 8, protein as a power food for brain concentration is different from an energy source). It is the preferred building block of muscle cells in your body. If you eat a skinless chicken breast, it is digested into amino acids, enters into your bloodstream, travels through your capillaries, and if your muscle needs it, will gain entry for muscle growth.

(Of course, if your body cells don't need the glucose and your muscle cells don't need the protein because you've overeaten, you know where they go . . .)

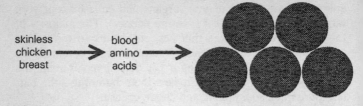

skinless chicken breast → blood amino acids →

**building blocks
for muscle cells**

Fat is not an efficient energy source for your cells or a building block of your muscle cells. Fat is efficient only at storing calories. Your body cells will use fat to function only if they absolutely have to.

If you eat a handful of cashews (which are mostly fat), they will be digested into triglycerides (a single fat molecule), enter into your bloodstream, and travel through your capillaries. They may go over to a brain cell, knocking on the door to gain entry, but your brain cell says, "Sorry, I'm not interested in you, but I'll take some of the glucose behind you." Then they may go over to a muscle cell knocking on the door, but your muscle cell says, "Sorry, I'm not interested in you either, but I'll take the amino acids behind you." The unwanted triglycerides travel through the capillaries to your fat cells and knock on the door. "We're so happy to see you. We've been waiting for you and have reserved your extra-large fat-cell suite. Come on in and make yourself comfortable."

If you feel sorry for fat, don't be too sympathetic, it is perfectly content with its storage role.

Are you convinced that the higher the fat content of your diet, the bigger your fat cells? I hope so because this final **OFF** strategy of fat-proofing your diet will add the finishing touches to help you outsmart your female fat cells. It will also provide a general feeling of well-being today and reduce your risk of disease tomorrow.

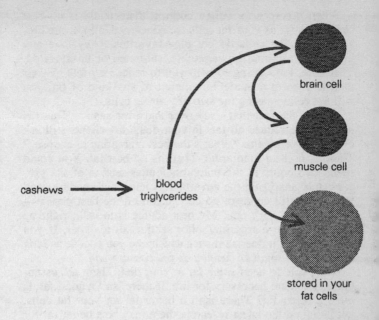

cashews → blood triglycerides

brain cell

muscle cell

stored in your fat cells

Reducing your fat intake is the single most important change you can make in your food choices. I could write an entire book on fat, its link to disease, the fat contents of foods, and the different types of fat, but I only have this chapter. I can sum up my message to you in one sentence: There really is no good fat. If it is not linked to heart disease, it's linked to cancer; and if it's not linked to heart disease or cancer, it will cause bigger fat cells.

If you are confused about fat, you are not alone. Our heads are spinning and we throw up our hands in defeat because we can't decide which fat to choose:

- Margarine or butter?
- Cream cheese or margarine?
- Lite cream cheese or regular cream cheese?
- Olive oil or corn oil?

When it comes to weight control, there really is no best choice. As far as your fat cells are concerned, all fats are created equal. Fat cells do not play favorites. They love any kind of fat: animal or vegetable, saturated or unsaturated. Therefore, I am going to help you to reduce *all* fats in your diet. If you eat a moderate amount of any kind of fat, you will not be increasing the size of your fat cells.

Despite the fact that I say over and over again: "There is no good fat; reduce all fats in your diet," my clients still ask over and over again: "What's the best margarine to choose?" There is no best margarine. There is no best fat. You could spend two hours in the margarine/butter section of the grocery store analyzing the advertising claims and reading food labels and still come to no conclusion on the best choice—because there isn't one. My best advice is to walk right by and ignore the margarine/butter section all together. If you must buy one, it doesn't matter which one you choose as long as you *use as small an amount as you possibly can.*

Now, you do need *some* fat in your diet. There are essential fats that are necessary for life. If there isn't a good fat, is there a better fat? There isn't a better fat for your fat cells, but based on the latest research, there may be a better fat for your heart. Olive oil has received the seal of approval for its favorable effects on blood cholesterol levels. Some people have taken this to mean that they can use as much as they want to and go through a bottle a week. Ten years ago, you were told to get rid of your olive oil. Today, you are told to use it. What are they going to tell us ten years from now? It's the good food/bad food cycle: What was bad for your yesterday is good for you today, and what was good for you yesterday is bad for your today.

My best advice is that when you need to use fat, use olive oil, but use as small an amount as you possibly can. That's my advice with any fat, olive oil or corn oil, butter or margarine. If you use a moderate amount of any type of fat, you are playing it safe for your fat cells and your health.

But what is a moderate amount of fat? How much fat should you eat a day? I could have you buy an expensive computerized dietary analysis program or go through a complicated mathematical equation to calculate the right amount of fat for you, but I won't. I dislike math probably more than you do, and would rather have you use that precious time and effort to continue making positive lifestyle changes and exercising.

Instead, I am going to share with you an easy, inexpensive, math-free way of estimating your fat intake. I want you to learn to balance your own fat intake. I call this the BYOF rule. It doesn't mean "bring your own fat," although it would make for an interesting party, it means:

B - Balance
Y - Your
O - Own
F - Fat

The goal is to choose foods throughout the day so that the average and balance over 24 hours is moderately low in fat.

So, to answer the question "What is a moderate amount of fat?" and "How much fat should I have in my diet?" my recommendation is that no more than 20 percent of your total daily calories come from fat. Your body uses calories to function—it doesn't use grams or ounces. Your body doesn't care how much a food weighs, it cares how many calories it is going to get from a food. And you have probably heard that fat provides more than twice as many calories as carbohydrates and proteins:

1 gram of fat	provides 9 calories
1 gram of carbohydrate	provides 4 calories
1 gram of protein	provides 4 calories

Gram for gram, ounce for ounce, pound for pound, fat is going to provide over twice the amount of calories. This is why I cannot give you a specific number of grams to eat a day. It all depends on the number of calories you eat a day· and that number is different for each and every one of you. Instead, I am going to show you how to estimate your percentage of calories from fat and how to achieve an overall 20 percent fat intake.

Depending on whom you ask, you may get varying recommendations on fat intake. Some experts recommend reducing fat to no more than 30 percent of the total calories; others to no more than 10 percent of the total calories. I recommend reducing fat to about 20 percent of the total calories. Here's why:

30 percent fat diet—is low enough to reduce your risk of disease and receive some weight-control benefit.

20 percent fat diet—is low enough to *significantly* reduce your risk of heart disease and cancer—and reduce your weight.

10 percent fat diet—is low enough to reduce your risk of all diseases and lose weight (and it's not so low that it will cause you harm)—but it is so low that it may cause feelings of restriction and deprivation.

Some people can follow a 10 percent fat diet successfully for the rest of their lives without feeling deprived. If you are one of them, keep up the good work. Other people, like me and most of my clients, do just fine on a 10 percent fat diet for about a month, then isolation and deprivation sets in. You can't go to restaurants. You can't go to parties. You can't have cake on your birthday. So in rebellion you say "to heck with this" and go from a 10 percent fat diet to a 50 percent fat diet. A 20 percent fat diet is the perfect middle ground. You will not feel deprived, but you will get all the benefits of reduced disease risk and reduced fat cell size.

To achieve a diet that is in the ballpark of about 20 percent of the calories from fat, all you have to do is ask yourself one important question: *Does the food I'm about to eat derive less that 20 percent of its calories from fat or more than 20 percent of its calories from fat?*

And balance your own fat intake with the BYOF "1 to 3

rule": For every food that derives over 20 percent of its calories from fat, choose at least three other foods that derive less than 20 percent of their calories from fat. Of course, if you didn't choose high-fat foods to begin with, you wouldn't have to balance your fat intake. However, most people do enjoy the taste of fat, so balancing your fat intake is necessary to achieve a low-fat diet. How do you know if a food derives less or more than 20 percent of its calories from fat? The following chart will give you a good start:

LOW IN FAT <20% CALORIES FROM FAT	HIGH IN FAT >20% CALORIES FROM FAT
Produce	
fruits and vegetables, fruit and vegetable juices, dried fruit, pickles, sauerkraut	olives, avocado, coconut, creamed vegetables, vegetable oils
Starches	
most breads and cereals, bagels, English muffins, pasta, noodles, rice, corn, barley, bulgur, oats, bran, potatoes, corn tortillas, rice cakes, pretzels, water crackers, air-popped popcorn, matzoh	muffins, biscuits, cornbread, waffles, pancakes, granola, croissants, pastries, donuts, flour tortillas, French fries, hash browns, snack chips, most snack crackers, oil-popped and micro-waved popcorn, wheat germ.
Dairy Products	
nonfat milk, nonfat dry milk, 1% low-fat milk, buttermilk, nonfat & low-fat yogurt, nonfat & low-fat frozen yogurt, nonfat and low-fat cottage cheese, ice milk, sherbert	whole milk, 2% low-fat milk, cream, half-and-half, whipped cream, ice cream, nondairy creamer, most cheeses, sour cream, cream cheese, creamed cottage cheese, butter

Protein Foods

halibut, cod, haddock, sole, flounder, red snapper, tuna, tuna in water, butterfish, shrimp, squid, clams, oysters, mussels, scallops, crab, white meat of poultry without skin, ham, Canadian bacon, pork loin, veal, round steak, flank steak, venison, rabbit, buffalo, egg whites, legumes

salmon, swordfish, shark, trout, mackerel, anchovies, sardines, dark meat of poultry, white meat of poultry with skin, most beef, most pork, most lamb, bacon, sausage, hot dogs, cold cuts, organ meats, nuts, seeds, refried beans, peanut butter, tofu, duck, eggs

Miscellaneous

broths, bouillon, most soups, spices, herbs, salsa, mustard, ketchup, horseradish, soy sauce, teriyaki sauce, vinegar, Worcestershire sauce, wine, fat-free salad dressings.

created soups, salad dressing, mayonnaise, margarine, oils, lard, beef tallow

Sugar Foods and Desserts

jam, jelly, apple butter, sugar, jelly beans, hard candies, licorice, lollipops, popsicles, fruit bars, sorbet, fig bars, animal crackers, ginger snaps, angel food cake, marshmallows, gelatin

chocolate, candy bars, most cookies, most cakes, pies, fudge, granola bars, tofutti, ice cream

If something is not on this list, you'll either have to do some calculations or make an educated guess. Most brand-name foods and processed foods have nutritional information on the package, which will allow you to figure out the percentage of calories from fat. All you need is the calories per serving and the grams of fat per serving. You already know that each gram of fat provides your body with 9 calories, so you first multiply the grams of fat by 9, then divide the total calories per serving to get the percentage of calories from fat.

grams of fat x *9 calories/gram* = % calories from fat
total calories per serving

Here is an example, if the food has:

> calories per serving: 150
> grams of fat: 6
> 6 grams of fat x 9 calories/gram = 54 fat calories
> *54 fat calories* = 36% of the calories from fat
> 150 total calories

(It's >20%, so it's high in fat.)

If there isn't any nutrition information on the package, your next strategy is to make an educated guess based on the list of ingredients. If one of the first three ingredients is a fat, then most likely the food is in the high-fat category. It may say "partially hydrogenated oils, corn oil, safflower oil, olive oil, palm oil, coconut oil, shortening, lard [yuck!], or butter." They are all pure fat.

Let's put the 1 to 3 rule into practice. It allows you to confidently balance your day's fat intake without driving you crazy. It doesn't mean that you can never eat a food that is greater than 20 percent fat for the rest of your life. That is not a realistic lifestyle change. Of course you will be eating some high-fat foods. All you have to do is acknowledge that the food is high in fat and balance it out by choosing at least three other foods that are low in fat. For example, if you are having salmon tonight for dinner, it's in the high-fat category. By eating the salmon, it doesn't mean that your entire meal has to be high in fat. You have the option of balancing out the meal with other low-fat foods.

> salmon   >20% fat
> rice   <20% fat
> broccoli   <20% fat
> nonfat milk <20% fat

Your meal is not going to be high in fat, it will be moderately low in fat because you balanced your meal with *three other low-fat foods*. But what if your entire meal is high in fat?

salmon	>20% fat
French fries	>20% fat
broccoli with cheese sauce	>20% fat
ice cream	>20% fat

This meal will not cause an immediate two-pound weight gain, clog your arteries, and multiply your cancer cells. It simply means that you ate a high-fat meal. So what? Have no fear: If this happens every now and then, then use the 1 to 3 rule: Balance your fat intake by making your *next three meals* low in fat.

BREAKFAST	LUNCH	DINNER
cereal	turkey sandwich	pork loin
nonfat milk	mustard	rice
juice	orange	carrots

What if you have an entire day that is high in fat? Maybe it is Superbowl Sunday or the Fourth of July or your birthday. Use the 1 to 3 rule again and make the *next three days low in fat*.

"I understand the 1 to 3 rule of balancing my fat intake, it's easy and realistic. But what if all of 1992 was high in fat? Do I have to make 1993, 1994, and 1995 all low in fat?" I answered yes and Cecilia's mouth dropped open. When someone teases me, I tease back. Needless to say, you don't need to go to that extreme.

The BYOF 1 to 3 rule is not exact; it is not based on amounts you eat, but it is an easy tool to estimate the fat content of your diet and achieve a lower fat diet. Because of its general nature, I need to alert you to one downfall of the 1 to 3 rule. I have had a couple of clients over the years get caught up in the numbers game of balancing their fat intake. For example, Sophie used this rule to rationalize every single high-fat food choice so that the end result was overeating. When she wanted a bagel with cream cheese for breakfast, she thought that she had to have two other low-fat foods with it to make sure her breakfast derived less than 20 percent of the calories from fat. She included cereal and nonfat milk (with the bagel that makes three low-fat foods), but now she was overeating and converting the cereal and milk to fat anyway to be stored in her fat cells. An even better example was when she wanted a chocolate bar for an afternoon snack. "I can eat it as long as I have three other low-fat snacks to dilute the fat content. So, I'll have some pretzels, rice cakes, and nonfat yogurt." She would have been better off eating just the chocolate bar and not overeating—then balancing her dinner with low-fat foods.

The message is not to overeat to balance your fat intake. High-fat foods may mean bigger fat cells, but so does overeating. Balance your meals and snacks when you can without overeating, but put more emphasis in balancing your overall day. Put a little cream cheese on your bagel or eat the chocolate bar, just make sure that at the end of the day you have three times as many low-fat choices as high-fat choices.

So you have the list of foods low (less than 20 percent) and high (more than 20 percent) in fat; you know how to calculate the fat content from food labels, and you are fully educated on the BYOF 1 to 3 rule and how to use it realistically without overeating. Despite all of this information, I still want you to beware of fat in disguise. As the saying goes, "There are two types of cockroaches in a restaurant: those that you see and those that you don't see." There are also two types of fat in foods: fat that you see and fat that you don't see. There are many foods that you may just assume are low in fat. Don't assume anything, do the calculations or look it up in a nutrition book—or put it on a paper towel and let it sit there for thirty minutes. You'll be surprised that certain crackers, snack items, breads, etc., leave a ring of soaked-up fat on the paper towel.

You may also be surprised what food preparation can do to the fat content of a food. A food may start out wonderfully low in fat, but how we cook it and what we add to it can make it a Mrs. Sprat's (you know, Jack's wife) delight. Here are a couple of shocking examples:

8% fat shrimp	deep fried	becomes 45% fat
7% fat cod	breaded and fried	becomes 62% fat
0% fat lettuce	with 1 tbsp of dressing	becomes 38% fat
5% fat bagel	with 2 tbsp of cream cheese	becomes 39% fat
0% fat zucchini	sautéed in 1 tbsp of oil	becomes 90% fat
0% fat berries	with 3 tbsp of cream	becomes 39% fat
0% fat pasta	with 1/2 c Alfredo sauce	becomes 54% fat
16% fat turkey sandwich	1 tbsp mayo	becomes 47% fat
0% fat potato	with 1 tbsp of butter	becomes 53% fat
	and 2 tbsp of sour cream	becomes 60% fat

There are many books available on low-fat cooking, and I encourage you to use them, but I would like to share six easy cooking techniques that will significantly reduce the fat content:

1. Use a good nonstick pan for sautéeing.
2. Use oil sprays, chicken broth, and wine for sautéeing.
3. Use fruit preserves in baking instead of margarine or butter.
4. Use evaporated skimmed milk instead of whole milk or cream.
5. Trim all meats before cooking and skim the fat after cooking.
6. Broil, grill, or bake instead of pan-frying or deep-frying.

There is one more technique that will help you to significantly reduce your fat intake. I want you to think about ten high-fat foods that you eat regularly. These foods are the major contributors of fat in your diet. It's not the French fries you eat once a month, it's the tortilla chips you eat every day. Over the next couple of weeks, experiment with low-fat substitutions that you like and find satisfying. Here's an example of a client's list to let you know what I mean:

HIGH-FAT FOOD	LOW-FAT SUBSTITUTION
margarine	jam
ice cream	nonfat frozen yogurt
potato chips	pretzels
peanuts	air-popped popcorn
bran muffin	bagel
snack crackers	water crackers
bacon	Canadian bacon
2% low-fat milk	1% low-fat milk
mayonnaise	mustard
olives	pickles

"But I have to have sour cream on my baked potato." Cindy tried every substitution, cottage cheese, nonfat yogurt, salsa—but nothing satisfied her as much as the sour cream. There may be certain high-fat foods that have no satisfactory low-fat substitutions. If you find that to be the case, use as small an amount as you possibly can. Satisfaction is very important.

PRIORITIZING YOUR FOOD CHOICES

Reducing your fat intake is the number-one priority in making food choices. And I have given you a wealth of information to make it a priority. However, past nutrition advice has focused on other criteria: We are told to choose foods that are high in fiber, low in salt, low in sugar, low in cholesterol. If you choose only those foods that fit all the criteria, you'd be living on whole grains and vegetables (fruits are high in sugar!), be hospitalized for anemia, and possibly die of protein malnutrition.

Fiber Choosing high-fiber foods will benefit your heart and your digestive system. I encourage you to include more fiber in your diet, but please choose low-fat fiber foods such as whole-grain breads and cereals, fruits, and vegetables. Bran muffins are my pet peeve. The whole country is eating high-fiber bran muffins in the morning. You walk into a bakery, scan the selections, consider the cheese puff, then say with confidence, "I'll take a bran muffin, please. I'm going to do my colon a favor today." Well, there is a lot more fat than there is fiber in that bran muffin—and the fat is not going to make your colon very happy. A low-fiber/high-fat diet has been linked to colon cancer.

Salt We have been bombarded with the no-salt recommendation for over twenty years. If someone catches you sneaking a shake on your food, you get the evil eye. We are not all sensitive to salt (as a matter of fact, only about 15 percent of us are), but we are all sensitive to fat. If everyone cut salt out of their diet, only about 15 percent of the population would experience a drop in blood pressure. I'm not telling you not to worry about salt (you may be one of the sensitive ones) or to eat a lot of salt—because it is still a strain on your kidneys—but to eat a moderate amount of salt and watch out for fat. I would rather see you eating salted pretzels than unsalted potato chips. I would rather see you adding salt to your potato than butter.

Sugar Many people have asked me, "Why have you included a list of low-fat sugar don'ts and desserts in your chart of the fat content of foods?" Because you have taste buds for sugar, and if you want a dessert or a cookie or something sweet, I would rather have you use the list to choose something low in fat than high in fat. Most foods that we consider "sugar foods" are actually higher in fat than they are in sugar. If you want a sweet fix, why increase your fat intake if you don't have to?

"You mean it is okay to eat sugar as long as it is low in fat?" many women ask in amazement. Well, yes and no. It's okay to eat sugar when you really want it, you are hungry, you enjoy every bite, and you don't overeat it. I'm not suggesting that you overeat sugar. I'm suggesting that when you want sugar, you choose low-fat sugar foods, and eat them when you are hungry. If you don't overeat it, sugar does not turn into fat in your body; and it is not linked to heart disease or cancer. And, contrary to popular belief, it is not linked to diabetes. A low-sugar diet is a treatment for diabetes; a high-sugar diet is not a cause of diabetes. The only proven link to sugar is cavities, so brush your teeth right after eating it. However, if you do overeat sugar, then it is converted to fat and it is linked to disease because it will cause you to gain weight.

Cholesterol We have been blinded not only by the no-salt and no-sugar recommendations—but also the no-cholesterol recommendation. Most people feel virtuous when they tell me, "I don't eat any red meat anymore. I gave up red meat two years ago because it is high in cholesterol." When I ask them what their protein choices are, their answers often include chicken legs, cheese, nuts, and salmon—which are as high, if not higher, in fat than red meat!

You don't have to give up red meat to achieve a 20 percent fat diet. You can if you want to, but you can also choose low-fat red meats like round and flank steaks. I know the message has been transmitted loud and clear: "DO NOT EAT RED MEAT," but the message we really want to get across is: "DO NOT EAT HIGH-FAT PROTEIN FOODS, NO MATTER WHAT COLOR THEY ARE."

It seems that with meats, what's most important is how you cook them. Broiling is better than frying, and the more well done it is, the more fat will drip out and the lower the fat content will be. So if you like you steak so rare that it could almost walk off your plate, it's going to be higher in fat.

And if you are still worried about cholesterol, you don't need to worry too much, as long as your diet is low in fat. Cholesterol is a problem only when your diet is high in fat. Let me take a moment to address the complicated cholesterol issue. We hear about cholesterol all the time, but do you really know what it is? Cholesterol is not fat; it's often described as a fatlike substance, but it really acts more like a nutrient in your body. Your cells, brain, and hormones need cholesterol to function, but you don't need to eat any cholesterol because your liver manufactures it. And, based on family history, some people's livers produce a lot of it.

Cholesterol in your diet becomes cholesterol in your blood only when it is in combination with saturated fat (animal foods, palm oil, coconut oil, and hydrogenated fats). If you choose low-fat foods and your diet is no greater than 20 percent fat, then the cholesterol in food will not be transported into your blood. Let me give you an example: Shrimp has the reputation of being loaded with cholesterol—and it is, but shrimp is also extremely low in fat. Shrimp alone will not have a significant effect on your blood cholesterol levels. However, if you deep fry it, or sauté it in butter, or eat it with French fries—it will definitely increase your blood cholesterol. You've added the saturated fat that transports the cholesterol into your blood.

Because of the heightened awareness of cholesterol and heart disease over the years (some call it hype), food marketing has focused on "no cholesterol" and "reduced cholesterol" claims. We think that the new, improved product is a good choice and throw it into our grocery cart—but a food can contain no cholesterol and be 100 percent fat. Many clients are buying low-cholesterol mayonnaise, cholesterol-free oil, and reduced-cholesterol snack crackers thinking they are also low in fat, but when they hear that the mayonnaise is 99 percent fat, the oil is 100 percent fat, and most snack crackers are 50 percent fat, they finally realize that cholesterol and fat do not necessarily go hand-in-hand.

Reduced-Fat Foods So the reduced-cholesterol claims might not mean much, but what about the "lite" foods or "reduced-fat" foods? They are a better choice, right? Not really. Don't be fooled, many of the "lite" foods are called lite because they are lighter in color and flavor or even simply because they are lighter in weight, not because they are lighter in fat. Most of the "reduced-fat" foods are made by taking the original food and adding water to it. Water contains no calories, so it just dilutes the fat and calories.

Since we are talking about reduced-fat foods, I'm going to use this opportunity to explain why food advertising claims are deceiving, particularly those foods that claim "95% fat free." You may think to yourself, "Wow! this is great. This food is only 5% fat," and throw it into your grocery cart. Most food companies evaluate the fat content based on weight, not based on calories. And, remember, your body doesn't care how much a food weighs; it cares how many calories it will get from the food. It is rather complicated to explain the difference between percentage of fat by weight and percentage of fat by calories, but let's give it a try.

This is an imaginary food, but most foods contain some fat, carbohydrates, protein, and water. This food has:

1 gram of fat	that provides	9 calories
1 gram of carbohydrates	that provides	4 calories
1 gram of protein	that provides	4 calories
1 gram of water	that provides	0 calories
4 grams total		17 calories total

If I were the president of this food company, it would be advantageous for me to evaluate the fat content of my food based on weight. There are 4 grams total and 1 gram from fat, so the food is 25 percent fat by weight. That is close to our less than 20 percent recommendation; however, the less then 20 percent recommendation is for percentage of fat by calories, not percentage of fat by weight. If we calculated the percentage of fat by calories, look what happens:

$$1 \text{ gram} \times 9 \text{ calories/gram} = 9/17 \text{ total calories} =$$
$$53\% \text{ of the calories from fat}$$

Now if, as the president again, I wanted to make this food a "lite" or "reduced-fat" version, I simply add water. Water adds weight to the food, but it doesn't add calories because water contains no calories.

1 gram of fat	that provides	9 calories
1 gram of carbohydrate	that provides	4 calories
1 gram of protein	that provides	4 calories
17 grams of water	that provides	0 calories
20 grams total		17 calories total

Look what has happened: The fat by weight has gone way down, but the fat by calories has stayed the same. There are now 20 grams total with 1 gram from fat, so the percentage of fat by weight is only 5 percent. The claim on this food could be "95% fat free." A true statement by weight, but not by calories. It still derives 53 percent of its calories from fat. Don't believe anything that you read on a food package— figure it out yourself.

Artificial Fats So that's the reality on many of the reduced-fat and fat-free foods, but what about the artificial fats? Just about everyone is asking me about them, so you may be wondering too. Are they harmful? Will they help me to reduce the fat content of my diet?"

There are a number of artificial fats that have either recently been approved or will be in the near future. To date, no harmful effects have been associated with them, but the question is what will we find ten years from now? They haven't been around long enough to analyze the long-term effects.

Now for the next question: Will they help? Some researchers think that they will help us to achieve a lower-fat diet, others feel that they will not have much impact. Again, it is too soon to tell, but if they follow suit with the artificial sweeteners, we probably won't see much benefit. Artificial sweeteners have been around for about forty years, and since then, our intake of sugar has increased slightly and so has our weight. It's only my opinion, but if Mother Nature didn't make it, our bodies probably weren't meant to eat it.

I want you to believe that it is important to eat a low-fat diet, but I don't want you to take it to the extreme. Some of my clients have what I call "lipohysteria." They try to make their diet 0 percent fat. They vow never to eat a food that contains fat. They vow never to feed their children a food that contains fat. Adults need some fat (about 5 percent of your total calories) to live. Children need more fat (at least 30 percent of their total calories) in their diets for brain and body development. You wouldn't want to compromise your life and your child's brain, would you?

To summarize, there are five fat-proofing concepts that have been addressed in this chapter. If you want to achieve a low-fat diet and smaller fat cells:

1. When you eat a high-fat food, eat as small an amount as you possibly can.
2. Balance your daily fat intake with the 1 to 3 rule.
3. Find satisfying low-fat substitutions for high-fat foods in your diet.
4. Prioritize your food choices with a low-fat content being the number-one criterion, and high fiber, low salt, low sugar, and low cholesterol being number two.
5. Beware of food advertising and nutrition claims.

Now that you have all the background to fat-proof your diet, let's put this final strategy into practice . . .

YOUR OFF ACTION PLAN: WEEKS 9 & 10

OFF Strategy Focus: Fat-Proof Your Diet
OFF Goals: 1. Continue with goals from weeks 1–8.
2. Reduce your total fat intake to 20 percent of calories by balancing your food choices.
3. Identify the fat content of foods by reading food labels and finding the hidden fat.

4. Exercise three times a week (four or five if you want) and increase the duration to 40 minutes each session.

OFF Techniques:

1. Remind yourself that there really is no good fat.
2. Practice the BYOF 1 to 3 rule for food choices, meals, and days.
3. Ask the important question: Does the food I'm about to eat derive less than 20 percent of its calories from fat or more than 20 percent of its calories from fat?
4. Use the fat-in-foods list.
5. Calculate the percentage of calories from fat using the nutrition information.
6. Estimate the fat content of foods by analyzing the list of ingredients.
7. Find satisfying and acceptable low-fat substitutions for ten high-fat foods that you eat regularly.
8. Use the hidden-fat test—put the food on a paper towel and let it sit for thirty minutes.
9. Add less fat to your foods.
10. Use lower-fat cooking methods.
11. Prioritize your food choices with low-fat content being number one and fiber, salt, sugar, and cholesterol being number two.
12. Broil or grill meats and cook medium to well.
13. Don't believe food advertising claims, figure out the fat content yourself.
14. **Keep food records for two weeks to practice these techniques.**

The food records for the final <u>OFF</u> strategy will still have you record when you are eating, your hunger level before eating, and your fullness after eating. But you will also assess whether each food choice derives less than or more than 20 percent of its calories from fat. Use all the information in this chapter: the fat-in-foods list, the food labels, and the ingredients lists. At the end of the day, you will total all of your less than 20 percent fat choices and all of your more than 20 percent fat choices. Using the 1 to 3 rule, you want at least three times as many low-fat as high-fat choices, or at least 75 percent of your food choices from the low-fat category. Here is an example:

THE FINAL FOOD RECORD:
FAT-PROOFING YOUR DIET

Time	Hunger Level	Approximate Amounts	<20% Fat?	>20% Fat?	Fullness Level
6:30am	4	english muffin	✓		5
		butter		✓	
		juice	✓		
9:30am	3	4 pretzels	✓		5
		nonfat milk	✓		
12:15pm	3	½ sandwich - ham	✓		5
		cheese		✓	
		mustard	✓		
		bread	✓		
		apple	✓		
3:30pm	4	½ sandwich - ham	✓		5
		cheese		✓	
		mustard	✓		
		bread	✓		
6:30pm	3	salmon - small piece		✓	5
		½ c rice	✓		
		½ c broccoli	✓		
		nonfat frozen yogurt	✓		
		TOTAL	14	4	
				× 3	

1 to 3 Rule: Are your >20% fat foods
× 3 less than your <20% foods? *Yes!* 14 12

If you have tried everything and still do not know the fat content of a food, make a guess. Your guess is as good as mine. Does it feel greasy? Does it taste like it is loaded with fat?

Here's the key question: Can you see yourself doing this a year from now? If you are trying to choose every single food at less than 20 percent fat, the answer is probably no. If you have made a firm commitment to yourself never to eat chocolate again because it is high in fat, how long to do think that will last?

Moderation and balance are what's most important to your eating habits and your fat intake. After a while, it will become second nature. You'll know which foods are high in fat and which are low in fat. You'll automatically balance your fat intake throughout the day. Use the blank food record on the following page as a guideline to start balancing your fat intake.

YOUR NEXT STEP IN AEROBICIZING YOUR FAT CELLS

Are your "next steps" becoming easier and easier? I hope so. That's the way it is supposed to work. You are already exercising three times a week; all you need to do is add a few more minutes to your exercise sessions. By the end of week 10, you'll be exercising three times a week for 40 minutes. Consider every minute after 30 minutes a fat-burning minute. That means 10 full minutes of maximum fat-burning exercise.

Of course, if the spirit moves you to exercise a fourth or fifth day, be my guest. But what's most important right now is the 40 minutes at moderate intensity.

THE FINAL FOOD RECORD:
FAT-PROOFING YOUR DIET

Time	Hunger Level	Approximate Amounts	<20% Fat?	>20% Fat?	Fullness Level
____	____	_____	____	____	____
____	____	_____	____	____	____
____	____	_____	____	____	____
____	____	_____	____	____	____
____	____	_____	____	____	____
____	____	_____	____	____	____
____	____	_____	____	____	____
____	____	_____	____	____	____
____	____	_____	____	____	____
____	____	_____	____	____	____
____	____	_____	____	____	____
____	____	_____	____	____	____
____	____	_____	____	____	____
____	____	_____	____	____	____
____	____	_____	____	____	____
____	____	_____	____	____	____
		TOTAL	____	____	
				× 3	
				____	

1 to 3 Rule: Are your >20% fat foods × 3 less than your <20% foods?

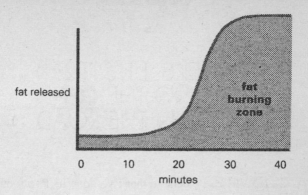

Remember:
- Stay in your moderate fat-burning zone.
- Sing "Old MacDonald."
- Schedule exercise on realistic days.

Chapter Eleven

■

WEEKS 11 & 12: TAKING THE **OFF** PLAN ON THE ROAD

"WOW! I can't believe that I've done it! I've focused on all six strategies, I've made changes in my exercise and eating habits, and I feel great. But now I'm a bit nervous—the holiday season is quickly approaching. For me, the holidays have always been a guaranteed fat-cell enlarger with parties, traveling out of town, relatives, eating out more—I've renamed the holiday season the 'pound-a-day' season. Last year I gained eleven pounds. What's going to happen to me this year?"

Maureen's nervousness didn't last long because she had the **OFF** Plan working in her favor. She didn't gain an ounce, and she still had fun. She took the **OFF** Plan with her everywhere—restaurants, friends' homes, relatives' homes, hotels, and even on airplanes. It had become so much a part of her life that she automatically followed the strategies during the holiday season.

Congratulations! You, too, have made positive changes with the 6 **OFF** strategies, and I want you to continue with all those strategies for this last two-week segment. I also want to give you the skills to take the **OFF** Plan "on the road" and use the strategies *realistically* (key word) during holidays, while dining out, and while on vacation.

At the end of this final two-week segment, you'll evaluate your overall progress in outsmarting your female fat cells. I realize that the mere word "evaluation" has some fear attached to it, "What if I failed?" You cannot fail the OFF Plan. You will not be graded, and you will not be compared to anyone else. There is no specific number of pounds or percentage body fat that you should have lost. The evaluation is only a tool to find out what you have accomplished and what you will accomplish in the future. Don't worry about the evaluation right now, I'll help you through it. First, let's address those food-focused, exercise-inhibiting special occasions where our attitudes and beliefs often sabotage our efforts. Do these rationalizations sound familiar?

"Well, Halloween only comes once a year."
"It's Valentine's Day, I'm supposed to eat chocolate."
"It's my birthday, I deserve my favorite cake."
"I'm on vacation from everything—including my exercise program."
"I have to clean my plate to get my money's worth at a restaurant."

It's perfectly natural to have these attitudes—every now and then. So what if you eat a little extra candy on Halloween, or have two pieces of your favorite cake on your birthday, or take a few days off from your exercise program while you are on vacation? The problem is that special occasions and the attitudes that go along with them occur more than every now and then. Holidays come at least monthly, and then, if you consider birthdays, anniversaries, and parties, special occasions occur weekly. Diane found an event to rationalize eating almost every day. "It's my cat's birthday, it's my friend's mother's birthday, it's payday, it's tax day, it's Friday."

Even if you don't search for special events to rationalize eating, there is always a holiday right around the corner. With the holidays coming so frequently and you giving yourself permission to overeat, your fat cells are going to have more of a celebration than you ever dreamed of having.

HOLIDAYS

An occasional holiday overindulgence will not sabotage your efforts and cause your fat cells to double their size. However, Thanksgiving to New Year's is not an occasional overindulgence. It can be five weeks of overindulgence. Is this a familiar situation?

It's Thanksgiving—what better reason do you need to overstuff yourself with thousands of calories. You are so stuffed that you have to undo your waist button and lie down on the couch for two hours. You've already blown it, so you have a turkey sandwich three hours later before bed and another one when you get out of bed the next day (usually starting with pumpkin pie for breakfast). Then you rationalize that it is only four weeks until Christmas with many parties and festivities—so why even bother to maintain anything that even comes close to control; you never have before. Before you know it, it's New Year's day, and you are making your resolution to lose the eight pounds that you gained since Thanksgiving.

By following the OFF Plan, you may not need any special guidance to make it through any holiday because you now have new attitudes and habits. But, if you are fearful of the holidays because of past weight gaining experiences and want to plan ahead to make sure that you survive the holidays, here are four *realistic* suggestions that will not sacrifice your enjoyment.

1. Don't Starve Yourself Overall, I would have to say that this is the most important strategy to help you maintain control. What do you usually eat on Thanksgiving Day? Most people have a slice of toast for breakfast and "save" the rest of their calories for the 4:00 P.M. feast. You are so famished by the time the appetizers make their appearance, that you devour them and are full before you even sit down to dinner. Then, by the time all the food has been passed around, your dinner plate looks like Mount Everest, and instead of climbing it, you eat it.

If you weren't starving before the feast, maybe you wouldn't have eaten as many of the appetizers or maybe your plate wouldn't look like a mountain range. Eat a reasonable breakfast and/or lunch and have a snack before eating to take the edge off.

2. Choose Special Holiday Foods My clients love this suggestion: Eat the foods that you really want and don't get very often. Why eat a little (or a lot) of everything else available when what you really want is the stuffing. Let me give you an example of what I do on Thanksgiving and Christmas. My favorite holiday foods are mashed potatoes, potato pancakes (my Aunt Gladys makes the best ones in the world—sorry Mom!), and kielbasa.

My family background is part Polish, so we have all the traditional holiday foods, plus an array of Polish cuisine. I used to have turkey, ham, salad, squash, bread, stuffing, mashed potatoes, potato pancakes, gravy, and kielbasa—and then go back for seconds on the potatoes and kielbasa. Now what I do is start off with the potatoes, kielbasa, and gravy, which is what I really want in the first place. Those are the foods that I have only a couple of times a year, and they are special to me and my family. I'm completely satisfied without feeling like an overstuffed turkey.

3. Balance Your Fat Intake If you follow the above recommendation of eating special holiday foods, your meal could be high in fat. Have no fear! The BYOF 1 to 3 rule is here. For the days surrounding the holiday, eat lower-fat meals so that the average for the week is going to be low in fat.

If you are making the holiday meal, then you can control the fat content. It's amazing what a few simple changes can do. Using a gravy separator will make low-fat gravy. Using evaporated skimmed milk in your mashed potatoes will make them low in fat. Choosing a fresh turkey will also reduce the fat content of your meal. Most turkeys are injected with fat.

Even if you are not making the holiday meal, you still have some control. You can choose the turkey breast over the leg, you can pass on the butter, you can put a small amount of gravy on your potatoes, you can bring an appetizer that is low in fat.

4. Exercise That Day Has it ever crossed your mind to exercise on Thanksgiving morning? With the OFF Plan a part of your life, maybe you will automatically schedule exercise into your holiday activities. Exercise helps you feel more in control and does burn a few extra calories. Many health clubs are open for at least part of the holiday. If you are unable to exercise that day, what about adding an extra exercise day that week? You may be eating a little more, so it wouldn't hurt to balance it out with a little more exercise.

After the feast, what about a family walk or another outdoor activity? "With my family? Are you kidding? The only movement they make is rising from the couch to walk into the kitchen for food—and that's strenuous activity for them." Lucy couldn't get her family to go for a walk, but *she* could still go for one.

Other holidays can present similar situations, but not as long or as intense as the Thanksgiving to New Year's season. Use these same strategies to help you through whatever holidays are difficult for you.

"I am truly amazed. This Valentine's Day I didn't eat two pounds of chocolate like I have the past ten years. I used to count the days to Valentine's Day because it was the only day of the year that I allowed myself to eat as much chocolate as I wanted to—and did I ever eat a lot of chocolate. This year I ate three pieces and that was it. I didn't want any more." The reason why Dorothy didn't want any more was because she was following the OFF Plan and had been eating chocolate whenever she wanted to. It wasn't special anymore.

Of course you can have chocolate on Valentine's, candy on Halloween, pumpkin pie on Thanksgiving, hot dogs on the Fourth of July. Depriving yourself of those foods is dieting: eat them when you are hungry (but not too hungry), don't overeat them, and balance your fat intake.

DINING OUT

Holidays present a problem for some of my clients, but dining out presents a problem for just about everyone. With the American public now spending about the same amount of money in restaurants as in grocery stores, we have to learn how to outsmart the female fat cell while dining out.

"When I go out to dinner, I always overeat. I feel so guilty afterward that guilty becomes my middle name." Lynne convinced herself that since the bread and butter were free, she should eat as much as she could. She also felt that she had to clean her plate to get her money's worth. If you share similar beliefs, let me give you some assistance.

The good news is that restaurants are beginning to get the hint that we want healthier, lower-fat food choices. There are salad bars and grilled chicken breast sandwiches at fast-food restaurants, some are serving the salad dressing on the side; some offer nonfat milk; some have a separate section of the menu dedicated to "heart healthy" or "lighter" entrées.

However, until restaurants really get the hint, you need to have a plan of action.

1. Ask Some Important Questions You have the right, you're paying for it. Ask how the food is prepared. How many times have you ordered a fish or chicken entrée thinking it would be a low-fat selection, but when it arrives it's swimming in a butter sauce?

2. Focus on Not Overeating As with the holidays, making sure that you are not famished may be the most important strategy to prevent overeating. The hungrier you are when you start eating, the more stuffed you are when you finish. To make sure that you are not overhungry, have a small snack before going to the restaurant to take the edge off.

Some other suggestions to prevent overeating include:

- Split an entrée.
- Order an appetizer as the main course.
- Order à la carte.
- Ask for a half order on pasta dishes and dinner salads.
- Ask that the foods you do not want be left off the plate (like chips and potato salad).
- Take the leftovers home with you.

Priscilla thought my next suggestion was ridiculous—until she tried it. She never left a restaurant before wiping her plate clean with a piece of bread. Leaving food on her plate didn't work, so I suggested that before she start eating she take half of what was on her plate and put it in a doggie bag. As long as it was off her plate, she didn't eat it. She still cleaned her plate, but there was half the amount of the food to begin with.

3. Balance Your Fat Intake If you really want the cheese omelet, have it—but choose a low-fat lunch and dinner that day. Ask for the dressing on the side. Ask for the vegetables to be prepared without butter. Order lower-fat meats, fish, and poultry that are broiled, grilled, or poached.

VACATION

Vacations can be double trouble. It's a special event, and it's usually dining out breakfast, lunch, and dinner. It's no wonder that most people gain weight while on vacation. You may lose weight before vacation because you always diet the month before departure, but then you gain the weight back plus an additional couple of pounds. You're sipping piña coladas, you're eating 9:00 P.M. dinners, and you're eating full-course lunches.

It may be impossible to lose weight while on vacation, but it is possible and realistic to *prevent* weight gain.

"I took the OFF Plan with me on vacation. I mean that I literally took it with me; I packed it in my suitcase beside my workout clothes." Every time Joyce opened her suitcase, it was there. It's what saved her from gaining her usual five pounds on her annual trip to Hawaii.

More and more people are going on fitness-oriented vacations: hiking, camping, biking, spas, wilderness camps. Don't automatically veto these and plan a trip to a remote island for twenty-four-hour relaxation. If you are not yet ready for a wilderness camp, at minimum choose a hotel that has an in-house gym, aerobic classes, and/or safe walking routes around town. When you do your research on accommodations, make this one of the criteria.

If you are a business traveler, your routine will be in continual flux. It is vital for you to make exercise a priority and schedule exercise into your appointment book before you go. There may be breakfast meetings, business luncheons, and dinner engagements—use the techniques for dining out and balance your fat intake. If your business plans call for air travel, you do have some choice in the meals offered. If you order a special meal in advance, you will be guaranteed that it is low in fat. From my experience, the seafood and fruit plates are the lowest in fat.

Let me summarize special occasions and events. They can still be special without an abundance of food and drink. There are four common strategies to follow whether it be holidays, dining out, vacations, or parties:

1. Don't let yourself get overhungry.
2. Choose those foods that are special for the occasion and that you really want.
3. Balance your fat intake and eating habits.
4. Stick to your exercise program.

Now that you have all the background to take the **OFF** Plan on the road, let's put this strategy into practice and evaluate your progress . . .

YOUR **OFF** ACTION PLAN:
WEEKS 11 & 12

OFF Strategy Focus: All Strategies: Taking the **OFF** Plan on the Road

OFF Goals:
1. Continue with goals from weeks 1–10.
2. Practice all the strategies together.
3. Practice the strategies during special occasions: holidays, dining out, vacations.
4. Exercise three times a week (four or five if you want) and increase the duration to 45 minutes each session.
5. Evaluate changes in your habits and attitudes.
6. Evaluate changes in your fat statistics.

OFF Techniques:

1. For these last two weeks, keep the final food record from chapter 10 in order to work on all strategies together.
2. Analyze your beliefs about food and special occasions.
3. Never be too hungry before a holiday meal, a restaurant meal, or a special event.
4. Have a small snack before the meal.
5. Eat those foods that are special for the occasion.
6. Balance your fat intake.
7. Choose lower-fat restaurant entrées.

8. Split an entrée, order à la carte, ask for a doggie bag.
9. Ask how the food is prepared.
10. Order special meals for air travel.
11. Pack your exercise clothes in your suitcase.
12. Choose a hotel that has a gym or exercise classes.

YOUR LAST STEP IN AEROBICIZING YOUR FAT CELLS

This last step will probably be the easiest in your exercise program. You are already exercising for 40 minutes at least three times a week; just add 5 minutes to each workout. That's 5 more minutes of pure fat-burning exercise, which makes a total of 15 fat-burning minutes! Since you began your exercise program in week 1, look how far you've come: You started exercising once a week for 10 to 15 minutes; now you'll be exercising three times a week for 45 minutes each session. That's an incredible accomplishment!
Remember:

• Stay in your moderate fat-burning zone.
• Sing "Old MacDonald" (if you are getting sick of this song, how about "Row, Row, Row Your Boat"?).
• Schedule exercise on realistic days.

EVALUATION

It is time to evaluate your progress. What successful changes have you made in your attitudes and habits? What successful changes have you made in your body fat, muscle mass, and body size?

There are two major purposes to evaluation:
1. To acknowledge your accomplishments.
2. To identify what you need to accomplish in the future.

"I don't think I want to do the evaluation. I don't think I can emotionally handle it if there isn't any change." This is a common reaction I get from clients when we get to this part of the program. Let me spend a moment preparing you for evaluation.

There is no denying that the stronger your commitment to exercise and the **OFF** eating strategies, the more change you will experience. But just as there are drastic differences between men and women, there are also differences among women. Two women may be following identical exercise programs, have the same amount of fat in their diets, and the same distribution of calories throughout the day—but experience very different changes in their bodies. The amount of change you will see depends on a variety of factors. Some of it may have to do with genetics, metabolic rates, past dieting practices, past pregnancies, and age. Some of it I cannot explain; no one can. It seems as if our bodies have their own mysterious schedule for losing fat.

If you have paralyzing evaluation fear while reading this paragraph, you needn't worry. If you have followed the **OFF** Plan, you will experience positive changes even if they are small changes. What we want to see is change in the right direction.

Just like everything else in this book, we are going to take the evaluation process slowly. First you will evaluate your changes in attitudes and habits in each of the **OFF** strategies. Next you will evaluate changes in your body composition and body size. Most women put the emphasis on how much their bodies have changed, how much fat they lost and muscle they gained. That is important, but I feel that your changes in attitudes and habits are even more important. If you have made great strides in the 6 strategies, your body will change. Even if you didn't lose a lot of body fat in the first three months, you will in the next three months. Those fat cells are stubborn—please have patience.

Let's evaluate your positive changes in attitude and habits. Back in Chapter 5 you filled in some questionnaires to assess your pre—OFF Plan attitudes and habits. I didn't tell you then, because I didn't want to bias your answers, but you are going to fill in those same questionnaires again. Without looking back at your previous answers (no cheating please), answer the questionnaires on the following pages, and then go back to Chapter 5 and compare your scores from three months ago.

STRATEGY #1: Have You Aerobicized Your Fat Cells?

Rate the following statements as follows:

0—Never, **1**—Seldom, **2**—Frequently, **3**—Always

	TODAY'S SCORE	PREVIOUS SCORE
1 I would rather diet than exercise		
2 I dislike exercise.		
3. I gain weight when I exercise		
4. I don't have time to exercise.		
5. I'll find any excuse not to exercise.		
6. I try to exercise, but I'm not consistent.		
7. I feel too fat to exercise.		
8. I exercise to the point of exhaustion.		
9. When I exercise, it's for less than 45 minutes.		
10. I exercise so that I can eat more.		
Totals		

How much have you changed?

STRATEGY #2: Have You Stopped Dieting and Started Eating?

Rate the following statements as follows:

0—Never, **1**—Seldom, **2**—Frequently, **3**—Always

	TODAY'S SCORE	PREVIOUS SCORE
1. I count calories.		
2. I'm either on a diet or off a diet.		
3. I eat diet foods.		
4. I feel out of control with food.		
5. Dieting is more important than good nutrition.		
6. I start my diets on Mondays.		
7. I eat for emotional reasons.		
8. Hunger is a foreign feeling to me.		
9. I wait until I'm extremely hungry before I eat.		
10. I eat to prevent hunger.		
Totals		

How much have you changed?

STRATEGY #3: Are You Feeding Your Body, Not Your Fat Cells?

Rate the following statements as follows:

0—Never, **1**—Seldom, **2**—Frequently, **3**—Always

	TODAY'S SCORE	PREVIOUS SCORE
1. I feel uncomfortably full after I eat.	_____	_____
2. I clean my plate.	_____	_____
3. I eat quickly.	_____	_____
4. I divide foods into two categories, "good" and "bad."	_____	_____
5. When I eat "bad" foods, I feel guilty.	_____	_____
6. I restrict "bad" foods and deprive myself.	_____	_____
7. If a food says "diet," I eat as much as I want.	_____	_____
8. I overeat healthful foods.	_____	_____
9. I overeat at restaurants and special events.	_____	_____
10. I eat standing up.	_____	_____
Totals	_____	_____

How much have you changed?

STRATEGY #4: Did You Shrink and Multiply Your Meals?

Rate the following statements as follows:

0—Never, **1**—Seldom, **2**—Frequently, **3**—Always

	TODAY'S SCORE	PREVIOUS SCORE
1. I skip breakfast.		
2. I skip lunch.		
3. I eat three balanced meals a day.		
4. I avoid snacking.		
5. When I snack, I choose "junk" foods.		
6. If I am going out to dinner, I eat little that day.		
7. I would rather eat food than throw it away.		
8. I feel uncomfortably full after lunch.		
9. I feel uncomfortably full after dinner.		
10. A meal includes meat, vegetable, starch, salad, and dessert.		
Totals		

How much have you changed?

STRATEGY #5: Have You Become a Daytime Eater?

Rate the following statements as follows:

0—Never, **1**—Seldom, **2**—Frequently, **3**—Always

	TODAY'S SCORE	PREVIOUS SCORE
1. I eat late at night.		
2. I eat before going to bed.		
3. I snack while watching TV at night.		
4. Dinner is my biggest meal of the day.		
5. I eat dinner after 6:00 P.M.		
6. I binge at night when I am alone.		
7. I raid the refrigerator in the middle of the night.		
8. I restrain my eating during the day, then overeat at night.		
9. The first thing I do when I get home from work or my day's activities is eat.		
10. Eating helps me to relax at night.		
Totals		

How much have you changed?

STRATEGY #6: Did You Fat-Proof Your Diet?

Rate the following statements as follows:

0—Never, **1**—Seldom, **2**—Frequently, **3**—Always

	TODAY'S SCORE	PREVIOUS SCORE
1. I love the taste of fat.		
2. I add butter or margarine to my food.		
3. I use oils in cooking.		
4. I put mayonnaise on my sandwiches.		
5. I eat out in fast-food restaurants.		
6. I eat deep-fried foods.		
7. When I read food labels, I look for the calorie content, not the fat content.		
8. I feel margarine is a better choice than butter.		
9. I'm more concerned about cholesterol than fat in my diet.		
10. If a food says "reduced fat," I buy it.		
Totals		

How much have you changed?

It's not only important to acknowledge positive changes in each of the strategies but also your overall accomplishment in the **OFF** Plan.

WHAT WERE YOUR SCORES?	TODAY'S SCORE	PREVIOUS SCORE
Strategy #1: Aerobicize Your Fat Cells	_____	_____
Strategy #2: Stop Dieting and Start Eating	_____	_____
Strategy #3: Feed Your Body, Not Your Fat Cells	_____	_____
Strategy #4: Shrink and Multiply Your Meals	_____	_____
Strategy #5: Become a Daytime Eater	_____	_____
Strategy #6: Balance Your Fat Intake	_____	_____
TOTAL SCORES	_____	_____
TOTAL CHANGE	_____	

Which strategies did you experience the most change in?
Which strategies did you still score above 15 points?
Which strategies do you still need to focus on?
List the Strategies From Highest to Lowest Score

1. _____
2. _____
3. _____
4. _____
5. _____
6. _____

It's important to quantify and measure your changes in the 6 <u>OFF</u> strategies. The goal is not to reduce every score to zero. If that is what you expected, it will never happen. Perfect scores and perfect eating habits do not exist in the real world. What we want to see is a reduction in points and to identify which strategies still need some additional commitment.

"My score for Strategy #3: Did You Feed Your Body, Not Your Fat Cells? was 28 three months ago and now it is 17. I really worked hard on this one and I thought I had done a good job, but my score is still above 15 points." You did a great job! You made positive changes that brought your score down 11 points. Change takes time; the higher your original score, the longer it will take you to change your habits.

For those strategies that are still above 15 points (or didn't change at all), read through the appropriate chapter again, set goals, keep the food records, and make a commitment to contained change.

Now it is time to evaluate changes in your body. The more positive change you made in your attitudes and habits, the more change you will see in your body. First, make an appointment to have your body composition analyzed again, and please stick with the same method. If you were underwater-weighed three months ago, get underwater-weighed again. Different methods can yield different results, and I want you to see changes in your body. Make an appointment with the same person, if possible. There is human error, so using the same person will help to minimize that error.

The only downfall of body composition analysis is that you have to get on the scale in order to calculate the pounds of fat lost and pounds of muscle gained. I know I told you to throw away your scale (you may have donated it to charity or burned it), but this is different. The only reason for hopping on the scale is to give you the whole picture on what has happened to your body composition.

Unfortunately, some women get caught up in the numbers. "What! I lost only five pounds, that's not even two pounds a month!" They get depressed even though they may have lost nine pounds of fat and gained four pounds of muscle. The scale brings back old feelings and the "diet mentality." I hope that after all the education in this book, it does not happen to you. If you think that you are not quite ready for the scale, you might consider what Paula did. She had the professional who was doing the body composition analysis blindfold her before she got on the scale and only got the final results.

What Has Happened to Your Fat Statistics

BODY COMPOSITION ANALYSIS	BASELINE RESULTS	TODAY'S RESULTS	CHANGE
Weight			
% Body Fat			
Pounds of Fat			
Pounds of Muscle			
BODY MEASUREMENTS			
Breast inches			
Waist inches			
Hip inches			
Thigh inches			

Besides the body composition analysis and body measurements, I also want you to notice general changes in your body:

- How much have your body measurements changed?
- Where have you lost the most inches?
- How do your clothes fit?
- Has your clothing size changed?
- How do you look in the mirror?
- How do you feel?

If you didn't see much change in your body, it's time to ask yourself some important questions:

- Did you fully prepare yourself for the program?
- Did you really take three full months?
- Were you really exercising three times a week?
- Were you really exercising for 45 consecutive minutes each session?
- Were you really exercising at a moderate intensity?
- Were you really listening to your hunger signals?
- Were you overeating?
- Were you eating more late at night?

- Were you eating for emotional and social reasons?
- Were you skipping meals?
- Were you eating high-fat foods?

Unless your ultimate goal was to lose only a couple pounds of body fat, it's not over yet. Three months is enough time to see some initial change in your body and provide the motivation for continued change. To reach your ultimate goal, read on. The last two chapters will give you what it takes to continue outsmarting your fat cells—and to outsmart them forever.

Chapter Twelve

■

AEROBICIZE YOUR FAT CELLS WITH A NEW ATTITUDE

"I NEVER thought that I would be admitting this, but I actually like exercising. In fact, I like it so much that I look forward to it. I've never been able to stick to an exercise program for three days, never mind three months. I'm not only doing it, I'm enjoying it. If I miss an exercise session, I just don't feel like myself."

Lucy was by far my most exercise-resistant client, so to hear her new exercise attitude was an incredible accomplishment. In our first session together, she walked into my office and announced, "I've never exercised in my entire life, and I have no plans to alter my anti-exercise behavior. Don't waste your breath talking to me about exercise." So, the word "exercise" did not escape my mouth for the first month. Then, as she became frustrated when her body barely budged despite changes in her eating habits, I started my exercise campaign. It was because of Lucy that I developed my "one small step at a time" exercise program: first committing to exercise just once a week for 10 to 15 minutes, then twice a week, and so on. If it worked for Lucy, it can work for any woman.

I hope that you, too, have experienced a similar new positive attitude toward exercise, because you are going to take this new attitude and use it to outsmart your female fat cells forever.

You may have thought that we were done discussing exercise. I discussed it in every single two-week segment of the

OFF Plan, and now I'm giving it its own chapter. What more can there be to say about exercise? There is a lot more to say about exercise because, as I have said before, *it is the single most important change women can make to outsmart their female fat cells*. I want you to fully understand how exercise changes your female physiology and how you can maximize your fat-burning potential.

Let's review what you have learned so far about your female physiology. Because you are a woman with estrogen, you were born a fat storer. The stubborn fat cells of your hips, buttocks, and thighs are continually fighting to survive and protect themselves with those lipolytic fat-storing enzymes. You already know that your fat-survival mechanism works most effectively when you diet. What about when you exercise?

Exercising, like dieting, can threaten your fat cells. They don't want to release fat, they want to store fat. When you start your exercise program, your fat cells say, "What? Release fat for energy? She's in Never-Never Land. Hasn't she realized that we are kamikaze fighters who will fight to the death for fat protection?" When a woman starts exercising, her female physiology starts working against her, and her fat cells start protection.

Women must be treated differently with regard to exercise. Women need special guidelines that will address their unique physiology and special needs. You have already started following some of those special guidelines in the 3-month OFF Plan:

You are exercising for a minimum of 45 minutes
at a very moderate intensity
at least three times a week.

By exercising 45 minutes at a moderate intensity three times a week, you have conditioned your stubborn fat cells to release fat and have shrunk your fat cells. This is the only type of exercise that will transform your fat-storing body into a fat-releasing body. It is the only way to stimulate the fat-releasing lipolytic enzymes.

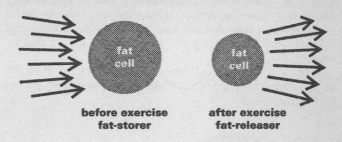

**before exercise
fat-storer**

**after exercise
fat-releaser**

If you haven't got the lipolytic enzymes, you are not going to release fat and shrink your fat cells. You can't buy them, you can't barter for them, you can't pray for them—you have to make them through exercise. This is not new, you've read it a number of times in this book. Now for the new information.

Once you've changed your fat physiology and released fat from your fat cell with the lipolytic enzymes, where does it go? What happens next? To become a true fat-burner, your muscle physiology also has to change. The released fat needs to be transported to a muscle cell, which is where the burning takes place. The fat cell's job is to store and release fat:

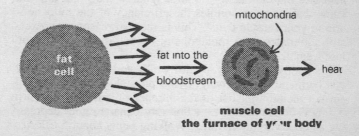

fat into the bloodstream

mitochondria

heat

**muscle cell
the furnace of your body**

the muscle cell's job is to burn it. The muscle cell contains important structures called the mitochondria that burn the fat and produce heat and water. The mitochondria are the energy centers of your body. It's like burning coal in a furnace or burning logs in a fireplace. You burn the fat in your muscles' mitochrondria. How much fat do you think your hair burns? Or your skin? Or your tonsils? *Your muscle mass is the furnace of your body.*

Without the muscle cell, the fat that you release from the fat cell during exercise wouldn't have any place to go, except back to the fat cell.

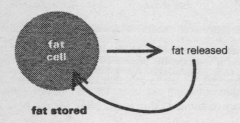

A woman's exercise program must focus on changing both her fat physiology and her muscle physiology. This is why an increase in muscle mass is beneficial for outsmarting your female fat cells. The more muscle you have, the more mitochondria you have, and the more fat you will burn. The bigger the furnace, the more heat will be produced. Exercise increases muscle mass (you already know that), but did you know that exercise doubles the efficiency of the mitochondria in your muscle cells? This is the real reason why exercise stimulates your metabolism, burns fat, and helps you lose weight.

It's not the calories you burn while working out, it's *what* you burn and *how* it changes your physiology. This is why I am not including a list of the number of calories you burn during different activities. I find those charts rather depressing and not very motivating. Walking burns about 5 calories a minute. So, if you walk for 45 minutes, you're burning 225 calories—that's not very impressive. It's the long-term benefits on your fat and muscle physiology that are impressive. Forget the number of calories you burn, and focus on changing your physiology and training your body to become a fat burner.

Let's compare men and women in their fat and muscle physiology. Maybe I should say let's compare the differences, because there are really few similarities. When a man starts exercising, his physiology works in his favor. When a woman starts exercising, her physiology works against her.

Men are born with all the ingredients for burning fat through exercise: more lipolytic enzymes, more muscle mass, and more mitochondria. Women are born with all the ingredients for storing fat: more lipogenic enzymes, less muscle mass, and less mitochondria. These are the reasons why men lose weight more quickly than women do and don't gain it back. These are the reasons why men immediately lose fat with any exercise program. They already have the lipolytic enzymes; they don't have to make them. They already have more muscle mass and more mitochondria; they don't have to make them. They have faster metabolisms and more fat-burning potential. Women can have that too, but they have to make it happen by changing their physiology through exercise.

Yolanda used to call herself a born loser, "but now I think I'll call myself a born storer." You may have been born a fat storer, but you can transform your body into a fat burner. The special exercise guidelines for women provide all the necessary ingredients for this transformation.

"With all these differences between men and women, wouldn't it be a heck of a lot easier to use steroids to change my fat and muscle physiology?" Sure it would. Women body builders who take steroids quickly increase their muscle mass and lose a lot of body fat. They also lose their femininity and fertility, not to mention the many other health hazards associated with steroids. The easiest way is not always the best way.

You need the lipolytic enzymes, the muscle mass, and the mitochondria. The process of fat burning for women also requires two other factors: oxygen and time. This is why I have stressed the importance of breathing at a moderate intensity for a long duration.

Let me put it all together so that you have a full understanding of the exercise-induced fat-burning process for women:

1. You need moderate exercise with a constant supply of oxygen to stimulate the lipolytic enzymes.
2. You need the lipolytic enzymes to release fat.
3. You need at least 45 minutes for the oxygen to stimulate the lipolytic enzymes and release a significant amount of fat.
4. You need to work your muscle mass to burn the fat that is released from the fat cell.
5. You need mitochondria and oxygen in your muscle mass to burn the fat.

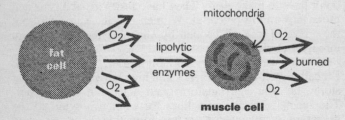

With exercise, you have provided all the ingredients: the lipolytic enzymes, the oxygen, the muscle, and the mitochondria. It's like making a cake: You need all the ingredients for the recipe to work. If you leave out one ingredient, the recipe just doesn't work. If you leave out one of the exercise ingredients, the fat-burning recipe won't work either. If you leave out the oxygen because you are working too hard, you won't burn fat. If you leave out the necessary time (45 minutes), you won't burn fat. They all work in tandem to transform your fat-storing body into a fat-burning body.

"All right already, I get it. Exercise is the secret to fat burning and outsmarting my female fat cells forever. I thought the secret would be a little less obvious and a little more original. Everyone recommends exercise." Everyone does recommend exercise and everyone has his or her own theory on the best way to exercise. The difference here is that I am recommending five specific fat-burning exercise guidelines designed for a woman's fat and muscle physiology.

If you have exercised in the past, you most likely have followed guidelines that were researched and designed for men—not for women. And you probably stopped exercising because the time spent resulted in minimal benefits. Exercise has been based on a man's physiology and cardiovascular system. Men can exercise for 15 to 20 minutes, and their fat cells will release fat. Men can also exercise at a higher intensity because they do not have the fat-protection mechanism for survival and have a more efficient oxygen delivery system in their bodies. Based on my experience, women cannot exercise as hard and must exercise for a longer duration to see comparable results.

If you are going to spend the time exercising, I want you to see the benefits with the five guidelines:

FAT-BURNING EXERCISE GUIDELINES FOR WOMEN

(aka: The Five Foolproof Female Fat Fighters)

1. Choose an aerobic, any aerobic, exercise. Remember, the type of aerobic exercise you choose doesn't matter as long as you follow the rest of the guidelines. All aerobic-type exercises are created equal because they use your major muscle groups (your buttocks and thighs) for nonstop, rhythmical movement. Walking is as good as running, which is as good as biking, which is as good as rowing, and so on.

2. Do it at a moderate intensity—never, ever, get out of breath. Because oxygen is involved in two steps, releasing fat from the fat cell and burning fat in the muscle cell, your rate of breathing and the delivery of oxygen are extremely important. Never, ever, get out of breath. Please remember this guideline and sing "Old MacDonald." Even if you are doing the same exact activity and one day you get out of breath, it's a sign that you are working too hard. Slow down. You may be walking at the same pace you always do, but if you are under a lot of stress or fighting an infection, it may be too hard for you on that particular day. Slow down so that your breathing and heart rate are steady and consistent. Your breathing has to be increased, but if you are huffing and puffing, it's too hard.

3. Do it a minimum of 45 minutes. If you want to be sure that you are releasing a significant amount of fat, then you must exercise in your moderate-intensity zone for 45 minutes. It takes 20 to 30 minutes to activate the lipogenic enzymes to release fat. Once they are activated, you have entered the fat-burning zone, so 45 minutes will ensure at least 15 minutes of fat-burning exercise.

4. Do it a minimum of three times a week. To see a significant change in your body, you need to exercise moderately for 45 minutes at least three times a week. Exercising once or twice a week is not enough to keep your body conditioned to release fat. Of course, you can exercise four or five times a week for even more benefit, but three times a week is the minimum at which you will still experience change.

5. Stimulate your muscle mass and mitochondria. Simply doing your aerobic activity will stimulate muscle mass and increase your mitochondria, but to change your muscle physiology even more, you may want to consider a light weight-training program. I'm not suggesting that you become a serious weight lifter, but if you want special focus on your muscle mass, consult an exercise physiologist who will design a program that is right for you.

These are the fabulous five exercise guidelines that have proved successful for my female clients. The problem is that most women and health professionals don't know that women need to be treated differently. *You* must be the one to make sure that your exercise program is providing all the ingredients. Laura was taking aerobics classes five times a week, but the hour class had only 25 minutes of true aerobic activity, the rest was warm-up, cool-down, stretching and toning. Twenty-five minutes was not enough time to activate her lipolytic enzymes to release fat. It was enough for her husband who was taking the classes with her, because he already had the enzymes and all the ingredients. When she viewed her exercise program as a way to change her physiology and increased her aerobic time to 45 minutes—she became a fat burner.

For a woman to lose body fat, she *must* follow all five guidelines. However, your fat cells are so smart and stubborn, that they may eventually figure out that you are trying to outsmart them with these special guidelines. You may need to continually keep your fat cells guessing.

"I've been walking for 45 minutes three times a week for about a year and a half now, and there were great changes in my body fat and weight until a couple of months ago. I haven't lost one molecule of fat in two months, but I want to lose more." If you find, which some women eventually do, that you have reached a plateau with your exercise program, it's time for an exercise boost to keep your fat cells guessing. If you do the same activity over and over again for the same amount of time on the same days, your fat cells will start to figure out what's going on. "Ah ha, it must be 5:30 P.M., she's pedaling again. I know how to do this."

If you need to keep your fat cells in confusion so that they will continue releasing fat—and you will continue seeing positive changes in your body—here are three exercise boosters:

1. *Add a few extra minutes.* If you were riding the bike for 45 minutes, make it 50 minutes.
2. *Add an extra day.* If you were biking three days a week, then add a fourth day.

3. *Add an extra activity.* If you were walking four days a week, then walk two days and bike two days.

Every additional minute is a fat-burning minute. Every additional day is a fat-burning day. Every additional activity is a fat-burning activity. Let me spend some time explaining this one. Each exercise uses different muscle fibers, so each stimulates different muscle cells to activate the mitochondria and burn fat. When you do the same activity over and over again, it becomes easier for you, so your muscle cells do not have to work as hard at burning fat for energy. If it is easy, your fat cells are not challenged enough to release fat. If you add a different activity, your body says, "Wait a minute, I'm not used to pedaling, I'm used to walking."

This is one of the reasons why cross-training has become popular. Instead of relying on one activity, you do two or more activities in your exercise program. You can either vary your activities on different days or vary activities in the same exercise session. This was the key for Cindi. She had been exercising for quite a while and had not experienced much change in her body. The day I suggested that she do three different activities in her 45-minute exercise session, she did it. When she went to her health club that night, she spent 15 minutes on the treadmill, 15 minutes on the bike, and 15 minutes on the stairclimber—and she lost more than 1 percent body fat in the next month! Her body never became accustomed to one particular movement.

If you need an exercise boost, add extra time, add an extra day, or add an extra activity. I'm not suggesting that you do all three, but, instead, do what is realistic for you. If you can't add additional time, add a fourth day. If you can't add a fourth day, then add 5 minutes. If you can't add additional time or a fourth day, then add a new activity.

My exercise recommendations have focused on changing your fat and muscle physiology. This doesn't mean that you can't play tennis, ski, golf, or go for a leisurely walk. On the contrary, I encourage you to use your new exercise attitude to become involved in many different activities. They may not be major fat burners, but they are fun and will stimulate your muscle mass. I also encourage you to move more in your day-to-day activities. You know how to move more on a daily basis; you don't need me to give you suggestions like take the stairs instead of the elevator. In our technological society, it has become too easy not to move. We have remote controls for just about everything. We have portable phones by our sides. We have timed coffeepots so we can sleep a few extra minutes. We have mail-order catalogs so we don't even have to go out shopping. These devices have been designed to save time and make life easy—they make life real easy for your fat cells.

Although my entire exercise guidelines have targeted aerobic activity to outsmart your female fat cells, there are two other components of overall fitness that I would like to briefly address: flexibility and strength. Flexibility is your ability to stretch your muscles. Some people are born more flexible than others (like the person who can place her foot over her head), but you can improve your flexibility at any age—and if you do, you'll have less injury and back problems and greater mobility. Stretching will help you to stay injury-free and is consistent with your aerobic exercise program. Consult with an exercise physiologist for proper stretching techniques, go to a stretching class, or join a yoga class.

Free weights, strength-training equipment, sit-ups, push-ups, and calisthenics will give you enhanced muscular strength and tone. These can and should be an important part of your exercise program, but let me share with you Tiffany's story. She was going to the gym four times a week for an hour and spending 15 minutes on the stationary bike and 45 minutes on weight training. When she made an appointment with me, she was ready to cancel her gym membership because she had gone from a size 12 to a size 14 in the last eight months. Her body got bigger because she had built a good deal of muscle mass from heavy weight training. That's great if your goal is to "bulk up," but it wasn't her goal. I told her to switch her exercise program around—spend 45 minutes on the stationary bike and 15 minutes on the weights. Why build muscle underneath the fat? You'll never see muscle definition unless you get rid of the fat first. After she lost body fat, she added more time to her weight program and toned her muscles.

As your new exercise attitude continues to grow, I have only one concern: that you not start exercising too much. Too much of anything can be negative, and that includes exercise. This may be the last possible thing you may think you'd overdo and be compulsive about, but some women are compulsive exercisers.

"I've been a compulsive dieter, a compulsive eater, a compulsive shopper—now I'm a compulsive exerciser. Me! The same person who said she hated exercise a year ago." Whether you are compulsive about it or not, if you overexercise, your body will be threatened and will stop burning fat. Too much exercise can make you a sugar burner instead of a fat burner; it can cause injury to your joints and muscles; and it can make you hungry and fatigued. You should never have to exercise more than five times a week for an hour, unless you're training for a marathon.

Because of the abundance of exercise misinformation from the media and from our friends, there are a number of common exercise misconceptions that I would like to address. These are the questions I am asked over and over again:

How can I spot reduce my thighs? If they haven't asked about their thighs, then it's their stomach or buttocks or hips. There is no such thing as spot reducing. A thousand leg lifts won't get rid of your thigh fat. A thousand sit-ups won't get rid of your abdominal fat. They may tone the muscle underneath the fat, but you will not see much change in your body. No matter what the popular fitness magazines lead you to believe, spot reducing doesn't work. The only way to get rid of fat anywhere on your body is through aerobic exercise. When you go out for a walk, fat will be released from all the fat cells in your body. Because you are a woman, the fat cells of your hips, buttocks, and thighs will be the most reluctant to release fat. But they will, even if it is at a snail's pace. All activities are fat reducing (and therefore spot reducing) over time.

How can I get rid of this cellulite? First of all, there is really no such thing as cellulite. Cellulite is fat. It is a term that someone outside of the medical profession came up with to describe the bumpy pockets that fat forms under the skin.

Have you ever heard a man complain of cellulite? Probably not, because the structure of their fat cells is a little different. No one knows why, but men have something that prevents their fat cells from collapsing and dimpling. It may be because they have thicker skin on the backs of their thighs, and, therefore, it doesn't show.

"I don't get it. Men have more muscle, more mitochondria, smaller fat cells, less fat, and now you are telling me that they also have less or no cellulite." I know, life isn't fair.

Although there are many over-the-counter remedies for cellulite, don't waste your money. The only remedy is exercise. Any cream that could dissolve the cellulite would dissolve your skin first. The wildest remedy I've come across is the Vacuum Pants; the claim was that they suck the cellulite out through your skin. If they were successful in sucking out the cellulite, they would suck out your blood vessels along with it!

What is the best time of day to exercise? On the same day, two clients read in the same paper about two different "best times" to exercise—and both their rationales make sense. "I read that morning is the best time because it boosts your metabolism for the rest of the day." "I heard that evenings are the best time because that's when your metabolism is starting to slow down and the exercise will give it a boost."

There is no best time to exercise as far as your metabolism and fat-burning potential are concerned. There is a best time for you: when it most realistically fits into your life.

Is it best to exercise before a meal or after a meal? Just like the time of day, the difference is insignificant. Some people claim that it is best to exercise before a meal because you'll be more likely to burn the calories when you eat. Others claim that it is best to exercise after a meal because you'll burn the calories you just ate instead of storing them. Both arguments have some validity. My conclusion is that it doesn't matter whether you exercise before a meal or after a meal. Exercising immediately after a meal is probably not a good idea because your blood supply is needed for digestion.

Is it true swimming is not the best exercise for losing fat? There have been articles in newspapers stating that swimming may not result in fat loss because the body's natural tendency in the water is to float—and fat is your flotation device. Fat floats and muscle sinks. Some also believe that fat helps to insulate your body in cold water. Intellectually this makes sense, but if you have fat to lose, you'll lose it swimming. For my clients who are convinced that swimming isn't a good exercise, I have them look at photos of Olympic swimmers. They may have a little more body fat than runners or bikers, but they are lean and fit.

What do you do for exercise? This isn't a misconception, but it is a question that just about everyone asks me, so you may be wondering too. I belong to a gym because I need it for motivation. I've tried working out in my home, but there were too many distractions. For me to do it, I need to pack my workout clothes and go somewhere with a fitness atmosphere. Also, for me to do it, I've discovered that I need some external stimulation to counteract the boredom (I'm no different from you; sometimes I find exercise boring too), so I either read (anything but a nutrition book and preferably a science-fiction novel or *People* magazine) or exercise in the TV room while watching my favorite program.

I spend about 50 minutes total, three times a week on the Lifecycle, Stairmaster, and free weights. Most people comment, "Only three times a week for 50 minutes?" My goal is to maintain not to lose more body fat. I've been exercising for fourteen years, and I am conditioned now and have reached my goals. When I feel my body needs it, I may add a fourth day or increase my duration to 60 minutes or so.

Can I say it one more time? Exercise is the only way to guarantee a permanent change in your fat and muscle physiology. *Exercise is the key to transforming your fat-storing body into a fat-burning body. Exercise is the most important strategy to outsmart your female fat cells.* Ninety percent of all people who have never had a weight problem exercise regularly—and 90 percent of all people who have lost weight and kept it off exercise regularly. What more can I say?

Chapter Thirteen

■

LIFELONG SMARTS FOR WEIGHT CONTROL

YOU MAY be thinking, "I've finished the 3-month **OFF** Plan. I've lost some fat, lost some inches, and gained some muscle. Now is the program over?" You've accomplished a great deal, but there are many more benefits to gain. It's far from over. This was not a three-month diet you just followed. With diets, you start on one day and end on another. With the **OFF** Plan, there is no end because the natural, realistic changes continue for a lifetime.

Let's reflect on your last three months. Before reading this book, you may have dieted, overeaten, skipped meals, eaten a lot late at night, eaten high-fat foods, and not moved a muscle. Your fat cells were switched on with powerful storage enzymes. This is probably what your fat cell looked like:

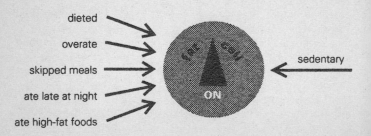

You had an abundance of storage enzymes and a deficiency of releasing enzymes. No wonder you couldn't lose weight—your fat physiology wouldn't let you.

After reading this book and following the **OFF** Plan for the last three months, you gave up dieting and are now eating a moderate amount of lower-fat foods frequently throughout the day when you are hungry. And you are exercising at least three times a week for 45 minutes. Your fat cells have been switched off with powerful releasing enzymes. This is what your fat cell looks like today:

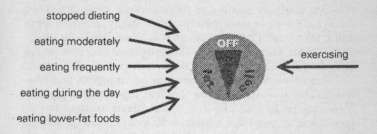

- stopped dieting
- eating moderately
- eating frequently
- eating during the day
- eating lower-fat foods
- exercising

You now have a deficiency of storage enzymes and an abundance of releasing enzymes. Because you have worked with your female physiology and followed the special eating and exercise guidelines designed specifically for women, you have finally switched your fat cells off and begun to see a permanent change in your body. *Lifelong smarts will keep your enzymes in balance so that you will continue to see permanent changes and shrink your fat cells forever.*

If you have reached your ultimate goals in three months, you either didn't have much body fat to lose, or you were a quick responder. Most likely, you have not reached your ultimate goals in three months, but you have changed your female fat physiology and have experienced initial changes in your body fat, muscle, and weight. This chapter will address lifelong smarts for continued change—for the next three months, the next year, the rest of your life. It will not take the rest of your life to reach your goals, unless, of course, they are unrealistic—in that case it will take you at least three lifetimes.

I want you to think of your future progress in 3-month steps. For the next three months:

- Which strategies are you going to target?
- How are you going to fit exercise into your schedule?
- If you are going on vacation, how are you going to take the OFF Plan on the road with you?

At the end of the next three months, schedule a body composition analysis again and monitor your progress. Then focus on the next three months. How many 3-month steps will it take you? That depends on you, your female fat physiology, your commitment to the program, and how much body fat you needed to lose in the first place.

There may come a time when you get impatient and frustrated. This is a slow process, but it is a permanent process. You may be tempted by a diet, but please overcome that temptation. If you have a friend who lost eighteen pounds in four weeks, instead of asking her what new diet she was on, ask her, "Eighteen pounds of what?" She will look at you with a puzzled expression, but you'll know that a lot of it was muscle and water. Then check in with her in a few months and see what has happened to her weight.

As your habits and body continue to change, please acknowledge those changes. We are sometimes so focused on the end result that we miss the important steps along the way. Give yourself credit, be proud of yourself, and reward yourself. Some of my clients have set up a reward system for continued motivation. Fran got a massage every time she lost 1 percent body fat. Kate bought a new outfit every time she made it through one month of exercising three times a week. If you like reward systems, then use one. Sometimes the positive changes in your body are enough of a reward.

Once you've reached your goals, then you need to maintain the changes and keep your body fit and healthy. In your past dieting endeavors, the easy part was losing the weight and the hard part was maintaining the weight loss. *With the* **OFF** Plan, maintenance is the easy part. It was a slow and committed process to lose the weight and body fat, but it will be easy to maintain the loss because you have changed your muscle and fat physiology with natural lifestyle changes. After a diet, your body wants to gain the weight back. *After the* **OFF** Plan, your body wants to keep the weight off.

Once you've reached your goals, I have only two concerns:

1. How you will accept (or not accept) your new body.
2. How you will adjust to life's changes.

ACCEPTING YOUR NEW BODY

"My goal was to get down to 24 percent body fat, and I'm there, but I don't know how much I like it. People are noticing me and complimenting me. It makes me feel uncomfortable. Everyone is telling me how terrific I look. If I look so terrific now, what did I look like before?" You may find that you attract more attention, that others find you attractive, that you feel more exposed. This makes some women feel so vulnerable and uncomfortable that it may cause them to gain the weight back so that they don't have to deal with it. Use the increased attention and compliments to make you feel good. Why not simply say "thank you"?

Some women may have difficulty accepting the social changes that go along with a new, fit body. Other women may not accept a new body because, in their mind, it is not good enough. "My goal was 25 percent body fat, and I'm there, but I still feel fat." So then they decide to get down to 22 percent body fat, then 20 percent body fat, then 18 percent body fat, and so on. Nothing they achieve is ever good enough. For some clients it has become their new obsession—it's always on their minds, it consumes their lives, and they have their body fat analyzed every other week. You never have to get below 25 percent body fat for health, and it is also unhealthy to get below 18 percent body fat. Women need more body fat than men. Women need about 18 percent body fat for all of the functions of womanhood. There is almost no limit for men; they can get down to about 3 percent body fat without compromising their health. Although some men may try, they can't get lower than that because there is essential body fat that is necessary for life. Part of that essential fat is in the brain, which is made primarily of fat. As soon as Donna heard this information, I could almost see the light bulb brighten: "So that's what has happened to my boss. In his pursuit of leanness, he has lost some of his brain."

Even though I have attempted to direct you away from the scale, some women still compare themselves to ideal weight charts striving to lose those last ten pounds. You may want to lose those last ten pounds, but your body may be perfectly happy and healthy right where it is.

I've known some women who have put their lives on hold until the scale hits that magical three-digit number. They are waiting for the scale to tell them "now you can be happy and get on with your life." Unfortunately, they may be waiting for the rest of their lives if their goals are unrealistic. Carmen had been waiting for eleven years—until she got smart. She came to the realization one day that her boss didn't weigh her in as a part of her yearly job evaluation to make sure she was at her ideal weight, and that her boyfriend didn't ask for a prenuptual weight agreement before they got married. She was the only one putting her life on hold.

It is very possible that when you reduce your body fat to 25 percent, you'll fall above your recommended ideal weight for your height. Many people who are lean and more muscular from exercise are told that they are overweight. Don't listen to anyone who compares you to the height/weight charts. As long as your body fat is 25 percent or less (but not less than 18 percent), you have found your own comfortable, ideal weight.

LIFE CHANGES

What if there has been an occurrence in your life that has caused you to stop exercising or to start overeating again? What if there has been an illness, injury, death, or tragedy that has taken all of your emotional and physical strength? An event may occur that will take priority in your life, and you may have to forget about the OFF Plan for a while. When you are ready and the time is right, get right back into it. Start with strategy #1 and integrate each strategy over the next three months. Your body will respond more quickly the second time.

The reason diets do not work is that they are unrealistic, temporary, and do not result in lifelong changes. The reason why the OFF Plan does work is because it is realistic and does result in lifelong changes. But life changes along the way.

Over the last three months, you have made lifestyle changes that are realistic and appropriate for your current lifestyle. But what is a realistic lifestyle change for you today may be unrealistic for you tomorrow. As a single woman in your twenties, maybe you could go to the gym five times a week and eat a small, early dinner. In your thirties and forties, with two children and a husband who works until 8:00 P.M., the gym and 5:00 P.M. dinners are out of the question.

As your life changes, your eating and exercise habits must change with you. The basics will always be the same: don't diet; listen to your body; eat moderate amounts when you are hungry; balance your fat intake; and exercise. It's *how* you achieve those basics that may have to change.

Not only may your lifestyle change, but your physiology may change as well. Fluctuations in estrogen will influence the physiology of your fat cells, and aging will influence your metabolism. I will take you through the major changes in a woman's life to help you make the OFF Plan work at every stage.

The Pill If you decide to go on birth control pills at some point in your reproductive years, you can expect the extra estrogen to cause a little extra body fat. The estrogen may stimulate more storage enzymes and make you a more efficient storer even when you are exercising and practicing positive eating habits.

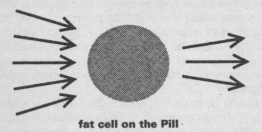

fat cell on the Pill

You need to balance your fat physiology by making more releasing enzymes. As you know all too well by now, the only way to make those enzymes is through your exercise program. Add a few minutes to your exercise session or add another day to enhance your fat-burning potential. The Pill will still cause you to store more fat, but the additional exercise will help you to release more fat so that you will not gain weight.

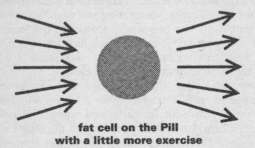

**fat cell on the Pill
with a little more exercise**

Pregnancy We've discussed the effects of pregnancy on female fat at various points in this book, but if you have never been pregnant, you probably skimmed over those paragraphs. If you do get pregnant at some time in the future please reread this section because you'll most likely have to outsmart your female fat cells again. The skyrocketing estrogen levels for nine months of pregnancy activates the lipogenic storage enzymes so effectively that it is difficult to deactivate them. This is a necessary physiological change for you and your developing child. There is no way to prevent it, and I don't want you to even think about trying. You and your baby need those extra enzymes and extra body fat.

During the pregnancy, continue with your healthy habits and your body will do what it needs to do for the pregnancy. By listening to your body's hunger signals, you will consume the extra calories that you need. You also need to gain weight and fat during the pregnancy, but some women gain more than is necessary. We've all heard (and maybe used) the excuse "I'm eating for two now" to give yourself permission to overeat without guilt. One of my pregnant clients took it to the extreme: "I'm eating for four just in case I have triplets." She didn't have triplets, but she gained about triple the amount of weight she needed to.

It's the time period after the pregnancy that I would like to address. Most women are told that if they breastfeed, they will lose the weight quickly and return to their prepregnancy weight. This works for some women, but recent research is disproving this breastfeeding/weight loss theory. There are many positive reasons to breastfeed, but weight loss may not be one of them. Women expect to lose weight quickly, and then if they either don't lose weight or lose it very slowly, they think that something is the matter with them. It's not you, it's your hormones. They are still at high levels during breastfeeding, and your fat cells do not want to release, they want to store. It goes back to that protective mechanism where your body wants to ensure plenty of stored calories for breastfeeding just in case famine hits.

Outsmarting your postpartum fat cells takes time. The storage enzymes need to be deactivated, and there are about ten pounds of fat that the body is reluctant to give up. Follow all of the strategies in the **OFF** Plan, be patient, and up your exercise program.

"I don't even have time to take a shower. How can I possibly find time to exercise with an infant?" If you want to see a change in your body, you have to somehow, someway find a place for exercise in your new life. If you can't arrange for a sitter or for your husband/partner to get home a little early so that you can make the aerobics class—then you need to use your imagination. I don't mean imagine yourself hiking up a mountain, I mean walk your child in a stroller or infant pack. Take your child on a bike ride. Ride a stationary bike while the child is napping.

I will not promise you that the **OFF** Plan will guarantee you'll get your prepregnancy body back. Pregnancy causes some women's bodies to change permanently: You may have loose skin on your stomach; your pelvic bone may be separated from delivery; if you had a cesarean section, your abdominal muscles may never get their strength and tone completely back. You will see positive changes, but they may not be complete changes.

Now, you may know someone who left the hospital as though she had never had a stomach the size of a beach ball. "I wore my size 8 jeans home from the hospital," your friend boastfully says. Don't compare yourself to her. She is the exception to the rule, a very unlikely exception to the rule.

Duel Career So now you've had a child (or two or three), and you are also working full-time. Even if you are a full-time mom without a full-time career, your mental and physical energies are directed elsewhere. With a full-time career on top of it, every waking moment is spent taking care of either family or job responsibilities. When are you going to find the time to take care of you?

This is very easy to say but very difficult to believe unless you've personally experienced it: If you take the time to take care of yourself, you'll be better able to take care of everyone and everything else in your life. You'll have more energy and be more productive. I told you it was easy for me to say—but it is true.

Some women are fortunate enough to have a sitter come to their home. Others have a close relative nearby to help. Others have a husband/partner who shares the responsibilities and lessens the load. Others do not have any means or luxury to make life a bit easier. Sandy was a single mother of three children, four, two, and six months old. She worked full-time for a salary that barely covered child-care. She didn't have any family members nearby and lived in the remote countryside. She couldn't afford a gym or additional babysitting. Normally, I would have recommended that she exercise at lunchtime, but she had only a thirty-minute lunch break. The only thing that worked for her was to exercise to an aerobics videotape at 8:00 P.M., after the kids had gone to bed. Do whatever is feasible for you to do.

- Join a gym that provides child-care.
- Take walks with your children.
- Join a neighborhood sitter's club where you trade off babysitting with other mothers.

Menopause Women comprise the greatest percentage of the population, and as a population we are growing older. Within the next ten years there will be more postmenopausal women than premenopausal women, yet there has been very little research on this major transition in a woman's life. This lack of research and attention is unfortunate and doesn't make much sense to me, but let me share with you what is known about the effects of menopause on the female fat cell.

Estrogen levels are significantly reduced, which may sound like a positive change because we have blamed estrogen many times in this book for our stubborn fat cells. You would think that when women enter menopause, they would lose weight because there is less estrogen to activate the lipogenic storage enzymes. However, most women gain weight, and some women gain a lot of weight without any changes in their habits. There is more to the physiological changes of menopause than meets the eye.

First of all, the reduction of estrogen levels means that ..ere will be more influence of the male hormone testosterone. This does not mean that you are manufacturing more testosterone and will become more masculine. It means that the testosterone that has always been present in your body will start to take effect, and your weight distribution will start to resemble the male "apple-shaped" pattern. All of a sudden women report that their pants and shirts are tighter in the waist. Or, as one woman put it, "My fat cells have migrated north during menopause."

Second, there is an overall 5 to 15 percent reduction in your metabolic rate. This means that even if your eating and exercise habits stay exactly the same, you will gain weight because your body's caloric needs are lower. And, because estrogen levels are lower, you'll most likely gain it in the upper body.

Now, what if you are a postmenopausal woman on estrogen replacement therapy? You will still experience the changes listed above. You'll have a reduction in metabolism and increased waist fat, but now you have some additional estrogen in your system that may activate the fat cells of the buttocks, hips, and thighs again. "Now I have active, stubborn, storing fat cells on every inch of my body instead of just the lower half."

Most women are confused about estrogen replacement therapy. Should I or shouldn't I take it? Most health professionals are confused too. I am not even going to attempt to give advice because it is beyond my expertise. However, if you (*you* are part of the decision!!) and your doctor have weighed the risks and benefits and have decided on estrogen replacement therapy, I want to make you aware of the physiological effects on your fat cells. A menopausal woman, whether or not she is on estrogen replacement therapy, usually has to focus on outsmarting her female fat cells once again.

"It's not fair. I've already outsmarted my female fat cells once before menopause. Why do I have to do it again? I thought life was supposed to get easier as I grew older?" Unfortunately there are always curve balls thrown at us, and life seldom gets easier. It's not as difficult as you may think to outsmart that mature menopausal fat cell. You'll use the same basic strategies of the OFF Plan with a little different emphasis.

Do not diet. Many women are tempted to diet to lose the weight that they quickly gained during the transition of menopause. You were not overeating, you were exercising—but you gained eight pounds almost overnight. The only thing a diet will do is slow your metabolism down even more.

Listen to your body. When your metabolism slows down, your body needs fewer calories to function. If you are truly listening to your body, you should find that your hunger and fullness signals will automatically adjust to your new caloric needs. You should find that you are hungry less often, and that you need to eat a little less food to feel comfortable.

Eat less at night. With a slower metabolism overall, you will experience an even greater drop in metabolism at night. Make your dinner meal as small as possible.

Fat-proof your diet. With lower estrogen levels, your risk of heart disease starts to climb. Estrogen protects against plaque formation in the arteries. You may need to reduce your fat intake even more to reduce your risk of heart disease and to reduce the storage of fat in your fat cells.

Exercise to boost your metabolism. I'm not going to recommend that you change your exercise program altogether, but I am going to recommend a couple of additions to your workout.

1. Add 5 to 10 minutes onto your exercise session. There is no way to completely prevent any additional fat storage, so add a few extra fat-burning minutes to balance it out.
2. Add a light weight training program. Women lose muscle mass as they grow older, and metabolism decreases with

the menopause. By starting a light weight training program with free weights or strength-training equipment, you will build and stimulate your muscle mass—and stimulate your metabolism.

3. Add three 5-minute intense metabolism boosters a day. Metabolism boosters are quick movements that increase your heart rate and stimulate your muscle mass. For example, doing jumping jacks or climbing stairs or jumping rope or running in place three times a day for 5 minutes would remind your body it is still alive and give your metabolism a boost. These are not enough to influence your fat physiology, but that is not their purpose.

Since we are discussing menopause, I would like to take this opportunity to address a major concern of menopausal women—osteoporosis. Why women wait until menopause to be concerned is baffling, because bone health is determined well before menopause. I'm not saying that there is nothing you can do about it if you are fifty or seventy years old, but if you are premenopausal, don't wait until menopause to be conscious of your calcium intake and bone health. If you are postmenopausal, you can prevent further bone loss and deposit bone to reverse the damage at any age.

What can you do to strengthen your bones? The answer to 99 percent of all health questions is—EXERCISE! You may be starting to resent the word "exercise." Is there anything that exercise doesn't do? Well, it doesn't help you to prevent athlete's foot, but that's about all it doesn't do.

You may have heard that weight-bearing exercise is beneficial for preventing and treating osteoporosis. This does not mean that you have to bench press 150 pounds; it means you have to make your bones carry your weight. Walking is one of the best weight-bearing exercises because you are making your bones carry your weight over a distance. With a stationary bike, the seat is carrying most of your weight. With swimming, the water is carrying most of your weight. Your bones have to carry your weight for it to be beneficial.

"Hmm, if your bones need to carry your weight to become

stronger, then the more weight your bones have to carry, the stronger they will become. So, is being overweight an effective preventive strategy for osteoporosis?" I had to answer yes to Muriel's question. She was looking for the one (and only) reason to stay overweight. If you are overweight, you are forcing your bones to carry your excess weight around every day. But that assumes that you do move your overweight body, and most women are overweight because they don't move. And, if you do move, the excess weight will be a strain on your heart, joints, and back.

Retirement "I was looking forward to retirement—more leisure, more travel, more time for me, but I didn't know that more weight came along with the package deal."

Retirement is a major lifestyle change. You are home more, you are around food more, you are traveling more, and you have more opportunities to eat. You may have more time to eat, but you also have more time to exercise. Use this opportunity to add an additional exercise day, take an exercise class, add some time to your morning walk.

Victoria used her retirement as the perfect opportunity to match her eating to her metabolism. When she was working, she barely had time for lunch and ate a large dinner. Now that she was retired, she had the time to switch her dinner and lunch around and make lunch the largest meal of the day.

No matter where you are in the span of life, life changes. Certain events in life either change your physiology, like pregnancy and menopause, or change your lifestyle, like marriage, children, and retirement. Use the information in this chapter to tailor the OFF Plan to your changing physiology, lifestyle, and changing needs.

A SERIOUS THOUGHT

It's just about the end of this book, and I think it's time to get serious. Not that I haven't been serious throughout the book;

I've been up front and honest, but in a lighthearted and up-beat manner. I'm not big on aversion therapy and fear tactics, but I think it's time to share some serious doom and gloom. Being overweight means disability and an early death. It may be from any of the weight-related diseases—heart disease, cancer, stroke, diabetes, gallbladder disease, or joint problems—but you will be robbed of years from your life.

The two leading causes of death for women are heart disease and breast cancer, and death rates are rising. A healthy lifestyle will be beneficial in reducing your risk of both of these diseases. If you are overweight and sedentary, you have about twice the risk of dying from a heart attack. By outsmarting your female fat cells, you can cut your risk in half.

Granted, there are no guarantees that losing weight today will prevent premature death tomorrow, but the chances are in your favor. A client gave me a T-shirt a couple of years ago that read, "Lose weight, eat right, exercise—and die anyway." It did make me laugh, and of course we will all die someday. But would you rather die sooner or later? Would you rather be healthy and active until the day you die or sick and bedridden?

You may have started reading this book wanting to lose weight for appearance, but I want to end this book knowing that you have also reduced your risk of many diseases and improved your health.

Lifelong smarts means accepting your new body; adjusting the **OFF** Plan to your changing physiological and lifestyle needs; recognizing your disease risk; and keeping all the **OFF** Plan strategies and skills a part of your life. There may come a time when you experience some low points and setbacks. If you do, read through these 25 statements that are the backbone of the **OFF** Plan. You've read them many times in this book, so reading them again may ignite the spark to get you back on track. If you feel that you need some personal support, consult with a registered dietitian—the expert in nutrition and weight control!

1. Forget the scale and have your body composition analyzed.
2. Forget the ideal body and find your own comfortable weight.
3. Think in terms of fat loss, not weight loss.
4. You can't starve a fat cell.
5. You have to eat to lose weight.
6. Work with your female physiology, not against it.
7. Eat what you want when you are hungry.
8. Don't let yourself get overhungry.
9. It's not what you eat, but how you eat it.
10. Get in touch with how your body feels with the hunger/fullness rating chart.
11. Any food is fattening, if you overeat it.
12. Eat mini-meals and maxi-snacks throughout the day.
13. Match your eating to your metabolism.
14. Make your dinner as early and as small as possible.
15. There really is no good fat when it comes to your fat cells.
16. Balance your fat intake.
17. Beware of food advertising.
18. Exercise is the most important strategy.
19. Transform your fat-storing body into a fat-burning body.
20. Never, ever, get out of breath.
21. Every additional exercise minute is a fat-burning minute.
22. Make only those changes that are realistic for you.
23. Tailor the **OFF** Plan to your specific needs.
24. The **OFF** Plan must change as your life changes.
25. Keep food records to monitor your progress.

Now you know everything that is known about female fat physiology. It may not have been what you wanted to hear, but it is the honest truth. A woman's physiology works against her efforts, and there is no magical solution to weight loss. But there is a realistic and permanent solution. *The* **OFF** *Plan works with the realities of a woman's body by changing the way her fat cells function.*

If you read through this entire book without following the **OFF** Plan, go back to Chapter 6 and make a commitment to start at the beginning with weeks 1 & 2. If you followed the **OFF** Plan for the last three months, I hope that you are 100 percent convinced that you *need* these eating and exercise strategies designed specifically for women to outsmart their female fat cells. *Without them, your fat cells are going to outsmart you.*

Now That You Have Read This Book . . .

■

A PERSONAL NOTE FROM THE AUTHOR

ISN'T IT about time that we viewed weight loss from the perspective of a woman's physiology? Isn't it about time that we developed eating and exercise guidelines specifically for women, based on their unique fat physiology? Through this book I have honestly attempted to piece together the puzzle of permanent weight loss for women. I have strived to raise social consciousness about dieting and the so-called ideal body. I have tried to provide the special attention you deserve to finally achieve success.

This book is not a fad diet. There are no gimmicks. There is no misinformation. There is no harmful advice. It is a natural, lifestyle approach that works with your unique female fat physiology. It is based on solid research, my professional experience with thousands of women, and my own personal experience.

I, too, have been influenced by society's pursuit of thinness, the diet mentality, and the stubborn female fat cell. I went through years of restrictive eating trying to find happiness in a thin body, only to find that thin is not synonymous with happiness. Even weighing close to 100 pounds (at five feet six inches), I still felt "fat." So, not being satisfied at 100 pounds, I turned to food for satisfaction and ate my way up the scale. No doubt, my own personal struggles influenced my career choice, and I became a nutritionist.

As a woman, I have come to my own conclusion that there

is no such thing as the perfect diet or the perfect body. As a nutritionist, I have had to come to terms with my body/food obsessions and have fostered a healthy relationship with food. I have learned that it is perfectly fine to be a nutritionist who loves pizza and potato chips. That it is okay to eat those foods when I want them. That it is okay to miss one of my scheduled exercise sessions. That it is okay to gain a few pounds premenstrually. Because my body is happy and healthy—and has been for the past eight years.

I believe everything I have shared with you in this book with all my heart. My only regret is that I could not personally help each and every one of you make this book a part of your life. As the next best thing, I have tried to be a coach, motivator, and educator through client experiences, physiological explanations, and personal insight. I hope that I have succeeded.

If I have made some small impact on your life, I have accomplished my goals. I sincerely hope that you have finally found success by reading this book—because it was written for you.

I wish you all the best in life.

Bibliography

■

SUGGESTED READING

American Heart Association Cookbook. 5th ed. New York: Times Books, 1991.

Bailey, C. *Fit or Fat Target Diet.* Boston: Houghton Mifflin, 1984.

———. *Fit or Fat Target Recipes.* Boston: Houghton Mifflin, 1986.

———. *Fit or Fat Woman.* Boston: Houghton Mifflin, 1989.

———. *Fit or Fat.* Boston: Houghton Mifflin, 1991.

Brody, J. *Jane Brody's Good Food Book.* New York: W.W. Norton, 1985.

Cannon, J. *Dieting Makes You Fat.* New York: Pocket Books, 1987.

Chernin, K. *The Hungry Self.* New York: Times Books, 1985.

Cooper, K. *Controlling Cholesterol.* New York: Bantam Books, 1988.

Goor, R. *Eater's Choice.* Boston: Houghton Mifflin, 1987.

Kano, S. *Making Peace with Food.* New York: Harper & Row, 1989.

Konner, L. *The Last 10 Pounds*. Stamford, Conn.: Long-meadow Press, 1991.

Hirschmann, J., and C. Hunter. *Overcoming Overeating*. New York: Fawcett Columbine, 1988.

Lambert-Lagacé, L. *The Nutrition Challenge for Women*. Palo Alto: Bull Publishing Co., 1990.

Lindsay, A., *The American Cancer Society Cookbook*. New York: Hearst Books, 1988.

Long, P. *The Nutritional Age of Women*. New York: Bantam Books, 1986.

Love, S. *Dr. Susan Love's Breast Book*. Reading, Mass.: Addison-Wesley, 1990.

Marano, H. *Style Is Not a Size*. New York: Bantam Books, 1991.

Nash, J. *Maximize Your Body Potential*. Palo Alto: Bull Publishing Co., 1986.

Orbach, S. *Fat Is a Feminist Issue*. New York: Berkeley Books, 1978.

Parker, V. *A Lowfat Lifeline for the 90's*. Lake Oswego, Ore.: LFL Associates, 1990.

Pennington, J. *Food Values of Portions Commonly Used*. New York: Harper Perennial, 1989.

Piscatella, J. *Choices for a Healthy Heart*. New York: Workman, 1987.

Roth, G. *Feeding the Hungry Heart*. New York: Bobbs-Merrill, 1982.

———. *Why Weight? A Guide to Compulsive Overeating*. New York: Plume Books, 1989.

———. *Breaking Free from Compulsive Overeating*. New York: Bobbs-Merrill, 1990.

———. *When Food Is Love*. New York: Dutton Books, 1991.

Satter, E. *How to Get Your Kids to Eat, But Not Too Much*. Palo Alto: Bull Publishing Co., 1988.

Schwartz, B. *Diets Still Don't Work*. New York: Breakthru Publishing, 1990.

Warshaw, H. *The Restaurant Companion*. Chicago: Surrey Books, 1990.

Weight Watchers. *Simply Light Cooking*. New York: New American Library, 1991.

REFERENCES AND SUPPORTING RESEARCH

Ailhaud, G. et al. 1991. Growth and differentiation of regional adipose tissue: Molecular and hormonal mechanisms, Int J Obesity, 2:87.

Alford, B. et al. 1991. The effects of variation in carbohydrates, protein, and fat content of the diet upon weight loss, blood values, and nutrient intake of adult obese women. J Am Diet Assoc, 90:534.

Bailor, D. et al. 1991. A meta-analysis of the factors affecting exercise-induced changes in body mass, fat mass and fat-free mass in males and females. Int J Obesity, 15:717.

Bjorntorp, P. 1991. Adipose tissue distribution and function. Int J Obesity, 2:67.

————. 1987. Classification of obese patients and complications related to the distribution of body fat. Am J Clin Nutr, 45:1120.

Brown, J. et al. 1992. Parity-related weight changes in women. Int J Obesity, 16:627.

Burgess, N., et al. 1991. Effects on very low calorie diets on body composition and resting metabolic rates in obese men and women. J Am Dietet Assoc, 91:430.

Campaigne, B. 1990. Body fat distribution in females: metabolic consequences and implications for weight loss. Med & Sci in Sports & Exer, 22:291.

Casimirri, F. et al. 1989. Interrelationships between body weight, body fat distribution and insulin in obese women before and after hypocaloric feeding and weight loss. Ann Nutr Med, 33:79.

Cauley, J. et al. 1989. The epidemiology of serum sex hormones in postmenopausal women. Am J Epid, 129:6:1120.

Coppack, S. et al. 1992. Adipose tissue metabolism in obesity: lipase action in vivo before and after a mixed meal. Met Clin & Exp, 41:264.

Cramps, F. et al. 1989. Lipolytic response of adipocytes to epinephrine in sedentary and exercise-trained subjects: sex related differences. Eur Appl Physiol, 59:249.

DenBesten, C. et al. 1988. Resting metabolic rate and diet-induced thermogenesis in abdominal and gluteo-femoral obese women before and after weight reduction. Am J Clin Nutr, 47:840.

Despres, J. et al. 1991. Loss of abdominal fat and metabolic response to exercise training in obese women. Am J Physio, 261:159.

Doolittle, M. et al. 1990. The response of lipoprotein lipase to feeding and fasting. J Biol Chem, 15:4570.

Drewnowski, A. et al., 1992. Taste responses and food preferences in obese women: effects of weight cycling. Int J Obesity, 16:639.

Eckel, R. et al. 1987. Weight reduction increases adipose tissue lipoprotein lipase responsiveness in obese woman. J Clin Invest, 80:992.

Freedman, D. et al. 1990. Body fat distribution and male/female differences in lipids and lipoproteins. Circulation, 81:1498.

Fried, S. et al. 1990. Nutrition-induced variations in responsiveness to insulin effects on lipoprotein lipase activity in isolated fat cells. J Nutr, 120: 1087.

Frisch, R. 1985. Fatness, menarche, and female fertility. Perspect Biol Med, 28:611.

Garrow, J. 1988. Is body fat distribution changed by dieting? Acta Med Scand, 723:199.

Geissler, C. et al. 1987. The daily metabolic rate of the post obese and the lean. Am J Clin Nutr, 45:914.

Haffner, S. et al. 1991. Increased upper body and overall adiposity is associated with decreased sex hormone binding globulin in postmenopausal women. Int J Obesity, 15:471.

Hattori, K. et al. 1991. Sex differences in the distribution of subcutaneous and internal fat. Hum Biol, 63:53.

Hirsch, J. et al. 1989. The fat cell. Med Clins of N Am, 73:83.

Hodgetts, V. et al. 1991. Factors controlling fat mobilization from human subcutaneous adipose during exercise. J Appl Physiol, 71:445.

Hudgins, L. et al. 1991. Changes in abdominal and gluteal adipose tissue fatty acid compositions in obese subjects after weight gain and weight loss. Am J Clin Nutr, 53:1372.

Jensen, M. et al. 1989. Influence of body fat distribution of free fatty acid metabolism in obesity. J Clin Invest, 83:1168.

Kay, S. et al. 1991. Associations of body mass and fat distribution with sex hormone concentrations in postmenopausal women. Int J Epid, 20:151.

Keim, N. et al. 1991. Physiological and biochemical variables associated with body fat loss in overweight women. Int J Obesity, 15:283.

Kern, P. et al. 1990. The effects of weight loss on the activity and expression of adipose tissue lipoprotein lipase in very obese subjects. N Engl J Med, 12:1053.

Kirschner, M. et al. 1991. Sex hormones metabolism in upper and lower body obesity. Int J Obesity, 2:101.

Krotkiewski, M. et al. 1983. Impact of obesity on metabolism in men and women. J. Clin Invest, 72:1150.

Lanska, D. 1985. A prospective study on body fat distribution and weight loss. Int J Obesity, 9:241.

Leibel, R. 1989. Physiological basis for the control of body fat distribution in humans. Annu Rev Nutr, 9:417.

Lindberg, U. et al. 1991. Effects of early pregnancy on regional adipose tissue metabolism. Horm Met Res, 23:25.

————. 1990. Regional adipose tissue metabolism in postmenopausal women after treatment with exogenous sex steroids. Horm Met Res, 22:345.

Litchfield, R. 1988. Oral contraceptives and fat patterning in young adult women. Hum Biol, 60:793.

Markman, B. 1989. Anatomy and physiology of adipose tissue. Clinics in Plastic Surgery. 16:235.

Martin, M. et al. 1991. Effect of body fat distribution on regional lipolysis in obesity. J Clin Invest, 88:609.

Mauriege, P. et al. 1990. Abdominal fat cell lipolysis, body fat distribution, and metabolic variables in premenopausal women. J Clin Endocrinol Met, 7:1028.

Miller, W. et al. 1990. Diet composition, energy intake, and exercise in relation to body fat in men and women. Am J Clin Nutr, 52:426.

Raison, J. et al. 1988. Regional differences in adipose tissue lipoprotein lipase in relation to body fat distribution and menopausal status in obese women. Int J Obesity, 12:465.

Rebuffe-Scrive, M. 1991. Neuroregulation of adipose tissue: molecular and hormonal mechanisms. Int J Obesity, 2:83.

————. 1985. Fat cell metabolism in different regions in women: the effect of the menstrual cycle, pregnancy, and lactation. J Clin Invest, 75:1973.

Rebuffe-Scrive, M. et al. 1983. Effect of local application of progesterone on human adipose tissue lipoprotein lipase. Horm Met Res, 15:566.

————. 1991. Effect of testosterone on abdominal adipose tissue in men. Int J Obesity, 15:791.

————. 1986. Metabolism of abdominal and femoral adipocytes in women before and after menopause. Metabolism, 9:792.

Rodin, J. et al. 1990. Weight cycling and fat distribution. Int J Obesity, 14:303.

Rosbell, Mr. et al. 1984. Effects of hormones on glucose metabolism and lipolysis. J. Biol Chem, 239:375.

Ryan, T. et al. 1989. Genesis of adipocytes. Clin Dermatology, 7:9.

Schultz, Y. et al. 1989. Failure of dietary fat intake to promote fat oxidation: a factor favoring the development of obesity. Am J Clin Nutr, 50:307.

Seidell, J. 1991. Environmental influences on regional fat distribution. Int J Obesity, 2:31.

Shimokatam, H. et al. 1989. Studies in the distribution of body fat: the effect of age, sex, and obesity. J Gerontol, 44:66.

————. 1989. Studies in the distribution of body fat: longitudinal effects of change in weight. Int J Obesity, 13:455

Simpson, E. 1989. Regulation of estrogen biosynthesis by human adipose cells. Endocrine Rev, 10:136.

Soler, J. et al. 1989. Association of body fat distribution with plasma lipids, lipoproteins, apolipoproteins in post-menopausal women. J Clin Edipdemiol, 41:1075.

Strokosch, G. et al. 1990. Lipoprotein lipase. N Engl J Med 15:477.

Tarui, S. et al. 1991. Viseral fat obesity: anthropological and pathophysiological aspects. Int J Obesity, 2:1.

Tonkelaer, I. et al. 1989. Factors influencing waist/hip ratio in randomly selected pre- and post-menopausal women. Int J Obesity, 13:817.

Tremblay, A. et al. 1989. Impact of dietary fat content and fat oxidation on energy intake in humans. Am J Clin Nutr, 49: 799.

Tryon, W. et al. 1992. Activity decreases as percentage over-weight increases. Int J Obesity, 16:591.

Vague, J. 1989. Sexual differentiation of the adipose tissue-muscle ratio: its metabolic consequences. Bull Acad Natl Med, 173:309.

Vansant, G. et al. 1988. Body fat distribution and the prognosis for weight reduction. Int J Obesity, 12:133.

Weststrate, J. et al 1990. Resting energy expenditure in women: the impact of obesity and body fat distribution. Metabolism, 39:11.

Wing, R. et al. 1992. Change in waist-hip ratio with weight loss and its association with change in cardiovascular risk factors. Am J Clin Nutr, 55:1086.

Yost, T. et al. 1992. Regional similarities in the metabolic regulation of adipose tissue lipoprotein lipase. Met Clin & Exp, 41:33.

Xuefan, X. et al. 1990. The effects of androgens on the regulation of lipolysis in adipose tissue precursor cells. Endocrinology, 126:1229.

Zamboni, M. et al. 1992. Body fat distribution in pre- and post-menopausal women: metabolic and anthropometric variables and their interrelationships. Int J Obesity 16:495.

Supplements To The <u>OFF</u> Plan

■

Seminars and Workshops

Debra Waterhouse is available for speaking engagements and training workshops. If your organization is interested in a presentation on "Outsmarting the Female Fat Cell" or other nutrition topics, please send inquiries to:

Debra Waterhouse
6114 LaSalle Avenue
Box #342
Oakland, CA 94611

Would You Like to Share Your Experiences?

If you would like to share your experiences with the <u>OFF</u> Plan, we would like to hear from you. Please include information on changes in the percent of body fat, inches lost, pounds of fat lost, pounds of muscle gained, and anything else you would like to share. Send comments to the above address.

The <u>OFF</u> Plan Personal Eating Journal

As a complement to the book, the <u>OFF</u> Plan Personal Eating Journal makes the important tool of record keeping simple, easy, and convenient. Small enough to fit into your purse or briefcase, it contains all the food records you need for the three-month <u>OFF</u> Plan—plus exercise records. To order this 100+ page "companion to success," please send $5.00 plus $2.00 shipping and handling to:

The <u>OFF</u> Plan
P.O. Box 4735
Portland, Maine 04112

Index

■